Advance Acclaim for

MINISTRY TO PERSONS WITH AIDS

"Robert Perelli's book is a timely addition to the AIDS literature. It brings family systems ideas to pastoral counseling. It provides important information and insights on spiritual issues for the nonreligious psychotherapist."

—JOHN PATTON, M.D.
Co-director, AIDS Project
Ackerman Institute for Family
Therapy and Research

"*Ministry to Persons with AIDS* is written for pastoral counselors and parish clergy with a background in counseling. It focuses on the crisis of AIDS in the male homosexual community and proposes that family systems theory provides a structure around which to shape pastoral counseling to people living with HIV disease.

"Robert Perelli examines the unique problems faced by gay men who are HIV positive or have been diagnosed with AIDS. Homophobia adds to the obstacles faced by this patient population, and Perelli emphasizes the need for counselors to be aware of their own needs and biases in caring for people living with AIDS.

"Dr. Perelli explicates Bowen's family systems theory constructs and explains how the theory may assist counselors in their counseling relationships. He concludes with a case study that illustrates how the theory may be applied."

—RONALD H. SUNDERLAND
Executive Director, Equipping
Laypeople for Ministry,
Houston, Texas

". . . a compassionate and careful analysis of AIDS as a family crisis, providing much needed insight for professional and volunteer caregivers to understand the effect of family patterns on the health of the person infected with HIV."

—CHRIS GLASER
Author of *Come Home!* and
Uncommon Calling

"It is good to have the family approach explored in assisting HIV + persons. . . . Perelli has contributed good insight—his distinction between 'spirituality' and 'religion' is a special necessity in dealing with persons caught in the HIV crisis. His work will help the caregivers dealing with the infected gay persons and their families."

—THE REVEREND CANON
EARL L. CONNER
President of the
Board of Directors
The Damien Center

"As a long-term survivor of AIDS, and being personally involved in providing pastoral care to those living with HIV infection, I know well the lack of material on the subject. Little has been written, and this is a positive, learned, and innovative approach to the issues."

—LOUIS J. TESCONI
Executive Director,
Damien Ministries
Washington, D.C.

". . . it was as if I was reading a narrative description of myself, how I felt, how I reacted, and how I panicked into a void of fear. . . . For me, an HIV + homosexual man, it was a mirror and an explanation of how Bob was helping me. These insights can be trusted. . . . To that member of the clergy who wants to help: Trust your compassion and rely on this information."

—"John," an HIV + man

GUIDES TO PASTORAL CARE

MINISTRY TO PERSONS WITH AIDS

A FAMILY SYSTEMS APPROACH

ROBERT J. PERELLI

Published in cooperation with
the College of Chaplains of the
American Protestant Health Association

AUGSBURG • MINNEAPOLIS

GUIDES TO PASTORAL CARE SERIES

*Ministry to Persons with AIDS:
A Family Systems Approach*
by Robert J. Perelli

*Ministry to Outpatients:
A New Challenge in Pastoral Care*
by Herbert Anderson, Lawrence E. Holst,
and Ronald J. Sunderland

Consulting Editors

Laurel Arthur Burton
Joan M. Hemenway
Arne Jessen

MINISTRY TO PERSONS WITH AIDS
A Family Systems Approach

Library of Congress Cataloging-in-Publication Data

Perelli, Robert J., 1949-
    Ministry to persons with AIDS: a family systems approach / Robert
J. Perelli.
        p. cm.
    Includes bibliographical references.
    ISBN 0-8066-2507-4 (alk. paper)
    1. AIDS (Disease)—Patients—Pastoral counseling of. 2. AIDS
(Disease)—Patients—Family relationships. 3. Family psychotherapy.
4. AIDS (Disease)—Religious aspects—Christianity. I. Title.
BV4460.7.P47   1991
259'.4—dc20   90-43093
                                                                CIP

The paper used in this publication meets the minimum requirements of American National Standard for Information Sciences—Permanence of Paper for Printed Library Materials, ANSI Z329.48-1984. ∞™

Manufactured in the U.S.A.   AF 9-2507

95   94   93   92   91   2   3   4   5   6   7   8   9   10

We humbly beg of you, O God,
  mercifully to look upon your people
  as we suffer from this dread disease.
Protect the healthy;
  calm the frightened;
  give courage to those in pain.
Grant to the dead everlasting life;
  console the bereaved.
Bless those who care for the sick,
  and hasten the discovery of a cure.

At this time, we remember especially:

Barbara	Marc	Kenneth
Paul	Thomas	Carolyn
Forrest	Jack	David Patrick
joey	Michael	Daniel
Brad	Phillip	William
Donald	Larry	Margaret
Gierald	Matthew	Dennis
David	Albert	Bonnie
Joseph	Victor	Scott

And finally, O Compassionate God,
  grant that in this and all our troubles
  we may put our whole trust and
  confidence in your steadfast love,
  through Jesus Christ, our Savior. Amen.

CONTENTS

GLOSSARY

ADC: AIDS Dementia Complex—most common neurological diagnosis in AIDS patients; marked by subtle cognitive behavior dysfunction that progresses to more severe dementia and psychomotor retardation (page 55).

AIDS: Acquired Immune Deficiency Syndrome—a disease characterized by the collapse of the body's natural immunity against disease. Because of this breakdown of the immune system, patients with AIDS are vulnerable to unusual infections or cancers that usually pose no threat to a person whose immune system is working normally.

AfrAIDS: Catchword for irrational and uninformed fear of being contaminated by the AIDS virus (page 19).

ARC: AIDS Related Complex (page 11).

AZT: Antiviral therapy that prevents some infections for people with AIDS (page 15).

Differentiation of self: The degree to which feelings and thoughts are fused—the central concept of Bowen's theory (page 58).

FWA: Family with AIDS (page 17).

Family systems therapy: A counseling methodology used to help a family with AIDS deal with the plethora of phychosocial stressors that accompany the illness (page 56).

HIV: Human Immunodeficiency Virus.

HIV +: Blood tests positive for antibody to Human Immunodeficiency Virus.

Homophobia: Total rejection of homosexuality as a normal and acceptable human choice about sexual orientation (page 17).

Homo-confusion: No strong views about homosexual behavior but confused by conflicting information available (pages 44–46).

Homo-negativism: Less outright attitude about homosexuals, choosing not to discriminate against or condemn, but will not accept someone in the family who practices (pages 44–46).

MAP: Mothers for AIDS Patients—organization that offers members services as substitute mothers for rejected AIDS patients (page 37).

PANIC: Prevent AIDS Now Initiative Committee—political extremist Lyndon LaRouche's organization to prevent infected people from certain jobs, etc. (page 48).

PHIV +: Person who tests positive for HIV (page 17).

PWA: Person with AIDS or people with AIDS (page 17).

PWARC: Person or people with AIDS Related Complex (page 17).

INTRODUCTION

At a time like this, when the crisis of AIDS is posing a threat to the physical and emotional health and welfare of modern society, the human family needs to rally its resources as it never has before in order to care for and counsel those afflicted with Acquired Immune Deficiency Syndrome (AIDS), AIDS Related Complex (ARC), or who test positive for the antibodies to the AIDS virus (HIV +) as well as prevent the spread of AIDS.

The focus of this book will be on the crisis of AIDS in the male homosexual community. Although some of the issues addressed are applicable to other people with AIDS, I also realize that extensive research must be done with the other groups whose behavior puts them at risk of infection, for example, IV drug users and their sexual partners, prostitutes, people who go to prostitutes, the urban poor (especially blacks and Hispanics) and young heterosexual adults with multiple sex partners. It is beyond the scope of this book to address those groups and their particular issues.

On a pastoral level the church has generally tried to respond compassionately to gay men and women. When it comes to the AIDS crisis, the church has sought to take a gentle and companionable approach to the needs of homosexual men suffering from the disease. However, many within the church interpret the

Bible and Christian doctrine to teach that the condition of being homosexual is "disordered" and the practice of homosexuality is immoral. This double message can produce confusion, anger, and rejection.

I became increasingly aware of this double message in my work that began almost exclusively on an academic level. A few initial appearances as a priest or counselor led to other invitations to speak on the role that the church always desires to play as a compassionate caregiver. The comments and questions were always the same: "Why is the church still so judgmental? Why do my wife and I feel like we are going against the church by loving our gay son? Why does it seem that the church can't say that we must love and care for persons with AIDS without the qualifier, 'While we do not approve of how they got AIDS?' "

My work eventually led me to establish AIDS Family Services in September 1989. AIDS Family Services provides psychotherapy in the family systems model to individuals, couples, and families affected by the Human Immunodeficiency Virus (HIV), as well as consultation, education, and pastoral care.

The crisis of AIDS may be one of the opportunities that helps the church to recover from what some have called "sexual bankruptcy" and become a better mirror of gospel values that cherish and respect each individual exactly the way God made him or her.

In order to address the issue, I will (a) point out the key role that the pastoral counselor or pastoral caregiver can play in ministry to persons with AIDS and their families; (b) identify and discuss the psychosocial stresses affecting persons with AIDS and their families; (c) describe family systems theory, which I think offers a particularly apt perspective for counseling people with AIDS; and (d) point out, with the help of a case study, how family systems theory can be useful in ministry to persons with AIDS and their families. The purpose of this description is not to make the reader into a psychotherapist but to open him or her to thinking systematically.

It is hoped that this book will contribute to improving the ministry and quality of pastoral care to people with AIDS.

Chapter 1

PASTORAL COUNSELING WITH THE PERSON WITH AIDS

When a person has AIDS the pastoral counselor or pastoral caregiver has a unique opportunity to interact with not only that person but the entire family. The church offers multiple points of entry into the family—probably more so than any other "system." In a large parish it is possible, if not probable, that the pastor will visit one grandparent in the hospital, bring communion to another grandparent every month, teach religious education to the junior high student, supervise the teenager in the youth group, marry the young adult, talk to the parents about a marriage problem, and preach to the entire family at a baptism, funeral, or (in some cases) every Sunday at church services. Few other professionals have as many opportunities to influence the family system at such significant times or with such regularity.

Based on the assumption that the pastoral counselor or caregiver has this entry into the family, it is fair to conclude that when a family is confronted with a crisis as devastating as AIDS, the pastor may be one of the most appropriate persons to help the family. "Because of long-term association that members of the clergy often have with a parishioner family, the appearance of a symptom in a child can be an unusual opportunity to gain entry into the entire family" (Friedman 1985, 101). In order to be effective in this position, the pastoral counselor or caregiver must be aware of certain facts about AIDS.

AIDS—Acquired Immune Deficiency Syndrome

AIDS is an "acquired" disease, that is to say, a person must "catch" the AIDS virus. Except for some children born of mothers who carry the Human Immunodeficiency Virus (HIV), people are not born with AIDS. AIDS attacks the immune system, the defense system that the body uses to fight diseases. AIDS is labeled "deficiency" because the immune system no longer works properly. It is called a "syndrome" because it is marked by a group of symptoms that affect different parts of the body.

AIDS is caused when the HIV invades the body's immune system and damages it in such a way that it can no longer ward off opportunistic diseases, that is, viruses, bacteria, fungi, protozoa, and carcinomas that take advantage of a weakened immune system. As the person's immune system becomes weaker and less able to protect the body from everyday attacks, the person moves from being infected—but healthy and asymptomatic—to being sick with a few more or less manageable symptoms, to being very sick.

At present, there is no definitive research to justify the common belief that all people who become infected with HIV will advance to the AIDS Related Complex (ARC) or AIDS or will die eventually. (A person with ARC does not have any opportunistic diseases, but begins to suffer from severe and persistent symptoms.) Although reports in the popular press have led many Americans to believe that the presence of the HIV antibody in a person's blood is a death sentence, statistics indicate that somewhere between 38 percent and 100 percent of such people progress to an advanced stage of the disease. With a 62 percent spread, this data hardy qualifies as definitive.

Presently, and for all the years that this disease has plagued our country, the largest group to be affected is gay and bisexual men. This statistic should not be construed to imply that only gay and bisexual men have to worry about this disease, or that gay and bisexual men are responsible for "creating" it.

Essentially, AIDS is not a matter of "being" anything; it is a matter of behavior. On the other hand, it would be naive not to recognize that, at least in this country, gay and bisexual men represent 58 percent of the cumulative number of males with AIDS. If the number of homosexual IV drug abusers is added to this statistic, the percentage of affected homosexual men rises to 64 percent. (These statistics are taken from the AIDS Weekly Surveillance Report, United States AIDS Program, Center for Infectious Diseases, Centers for Disease Control, February 1990, see the chart on p. 16.) In the past, that statistic has been as high as 74 percent. These facts demand that we maintain a delicate balance between the fact that *everyone* is vulnerable to AIDS and that, at this point in the history of AIDS, we need to focus special attention on the gay and bisexual community.

Currently, prevention is the best defense against this rapidly spreading disease. In order to understand prevention, we must first understand transmission. HIV is transmitted by blood-to-blood or semen-to-blood contact. Consequently, the primary modes of transmission for the AIDS virus are (1) sexual contact involving an exchange of blood or semen; (2) the sharing of intravenous needles among IV drug users; (3) from mother to infant (while in utero, during the birth process, or via breast milk); and (4) prior to 1985, by the transfusion of infected blood or blood products. While the key modes of transmission are related to body fluids, not all body fluids are transmitters of HIV. It is important to note that the general public has nothing to fear from saliva, tears, or sweat. The proverb "an ounce of prevention is worth a pound of cure" applies to the AIDS crisis. The only "cure" for AIDS is making sure no one else gets it.

As of yet there is no remedy for AIDS and scientists speculate that a vaccine to prevent AIDS virus infection is more likely than a medication to cure a person who is infected. Consequently, for people who are already infected, much research revolves around treatments to ward off the opportunistic infections that are usually the cause of death. At the present time AZT is an antiviral therapy that prevents some opportunistic infections in many people with AIDS (PWAs) and people with ARC (PWARCs). For our purpose it is enough to recognize that, at this point, the best defense is to maintain the health of the person with AIDS (PWA), the person

Adult/adolescent AIDS cases by single and multiple exposure categories, reported through February 1990, United States

Exposure category	AIDS cases	
	No.	(%)
Single mode of exposure		
Male homosexual/bisexual contact	71,026	(58)
Intravenous (IV) drug use (female and heterosexual male)	22,332	(18)
Hemophilia/coagulation disorder	668	(1)
Heterosexual contact	5,737	(5)
Receipt of transfusion of blood, blood component, or tissue	2,984	(2)
Other/undetermined	4,131	(3)
Single mode of exposure subtotal	**106,878**	**(87)**
Multiple modes of exposure		
Male homosexual/bisexual contact; IV drug use	7,707	(6)
Male homosexual/bisexual contact; hemophilia	27	(0)
Male homosexual/bisexual contact; heterosexual contact	1,441	(1)
Male homosexual/bisexual contact; receipt of transfusion	1,400	(1)
IV drug use; hemophilia	30	(0)
IV drug use; heterosexual contact	2,933	(2)
IV drug use; receipt of transfusion	602	(0)
Hemophilia; heterosexual contact	5	(0)
Hemophilia; receipt of transfusion	432	(0)
Heterosexual contact; receipt of transfusion	290	(0)
Male homosexual/bisexual contact; IV drug use; hemophilia	11	(0)
Male homosexual/bisexual contact; IV drug use; heterosexual contact	548	(0)
Male homosexual/bisexual contact; IV drug use; receipt of transfusion	229	(0)
Male homosexual/bisexual contact; hemophilia; heterosexual contact	2	(0)
Male homosexual/bisexual contact; hemophilia; receipt of transfusion	17	(0)
Male homosexual/bisexual contact; heterosexual contact; receipt of transfusion	77	(0)
IV drug use; hemophilia; heterosexual contact	4	(0)
IV drug use; hemophilia; receipt of transfusion	17	(0)
IV drug use; heterosexual contact; receipt of transfusion	169	(0)
Hemophilia; heterosexual contact; receipt of transfusion	9	(0)
Male homosexual/bisexual contact; IV drug use; hemophilia; receipt of transfusion	8	(0)
Male homosexual/bisexual contact; IV drug use; heterosexual contact; receipt of transfusion	27	(0)
IV drug use; hemophilia; heterosexual contact; receipt of transfusion	5	(0)
Multiple modes of exposure subtotal	**15,990**	**(13)**
Total	**122,868**	**(100)**

with ARC (PWARC), and the person who tests HIV positive (PHIV+) in an effort to prevent (for the PHIV+) or postpone (for the PWARC and PWA) the weakening of his or her immune system and the onslaught of opportunistic diseases.

The Person of the Therapist

He stuck his head in the door. When I saw he was a priest, I began to cry because I was hoping to reconcile myself with the Church. But the priest did not understand my tears. He seemed to panic and began to repeat again and again, "Don't cry, please don't cry." I tried to explain, but he was not able to hear. He told me what time Mass was and left in a rush. I doubt I could have talked to him. He seemed to be afraid of me (Flynn 1986, 57).

Before working with families or persons with AIDS, the pastoral counselor or caregiver must deal with his or her own fears. Those fears may include homophobia, fear of death, or fear of contamination.

Homophobia has been documented as a major obstacle in the medical care of PWAs. It would not be hard to extrapolate that it also an impediment to their pastoral care. If a pastoral counselor or caregiver has unresolved attitudes about his or her sexuality, it would be easy for him or her to project those feelings onto a gay PWA. This projection might take the form of a refusal to visit the PWA parishioner while he was hospitalized, a cold attitude in any interaction with the PWA and FWA (families with AIDS), or even a belief that the pastoral counselor or caregiver must "convert" the PWA from homosexuality or convince him to renounce his lover before his death. Such attitudes are inappropriate and dangerous. However, recognition of these feelings could be an excellent opportunity for the pastoral counselor or caregiver to assume the position of the "wounded healer" and take a deeper look at his or her own attitudes about sexuality. Pastoral counseling and care to PWAs might be one of those wonderful situations when the one being ministered to turns out to be the one who is doing the real ministry.

There are initially only two kinds of people: Those who sin and those who are not truly tempted. Many are spared certain temptations because some aspects of their human nature (such as righteous wrath and a healthy sensuality) are frozen and have never thawed enough to be either blessings or problems. So in many cases "We atone for the sins that we're most inclined to, by condemning the ones that we have no mind to." (Gallagher 1987, 8).

Some pastors may feel uneasy dealing with the gay PWA because of the conflict between the theology of pastoral care of the sick and the teaching on homosexuality and homosexual activity. These people can be reinforced in their ministry if they take to heart the church's teaching about Jesus' compassion and forgiveness. This is not to imply that the gay PWA needs to be forgiven for being gay, but rather that the pastoral counselor or caregiver needs to accept the gay PWA at whatever point he is at in his journey of faith—a journey that almost always includes a walk with forgiveness.

Once pastoral counselors or caregivers can face their own homophobia, they will need to be courageous because criticism for working with PWAs will probably follow. People will question the clergyperson's sexual orientation, motives, and orthodoxy. That is one way people project their own homophobia on others. Pastoral counselors or caregivers would be naive not to take this into consideration before they begin a public ministry to the PWA and FWA. Equally naive would be the minister who entered this field without a support system of other people who minister to the PWA and FWA, or without superiors and family members who are understanding, accepting, and supportive (Shelp and Sunderland 1987, 93–94).

Pastoral counselors or caregivers also need to face their fear of serious illness and death. AIDS can be a horrible death to witness. One never knows the course that it will take: wasting, dementia, severe pain, long and repeated hospitalizations, an almost incomprehensible sense of loss and grief, an ever-increasing need for care often ending with the need for round-the-clock attention. Caregivers must be aware of all these possibilities and anticipate their own needs so that they will be capable of walking with the FWA on this often long and painful journey. The pastoral counselor may need a supportive environment where he or she can process the feelings that come from watching young men die in their prime. This supportive environment could take the form of a personal therapist or a support group of other professionals from the field. Either way, it would be to the minister's advantage to build some form of support into his or her work with the FWA.

The lack of true knowledge about the spread of AIDS can be one of the most powerful contributors to the spread of "Afr-AIDS." "AfrAIDS" is the catchword for the irrational and un-informed fear of being contaminated by the AIDS virus. Even the medical profession, with all its knowledge about epidemiology and its techniques for isolation, is not exempt from irrational fears of contracting AIDS. The pastoral counselor or caregiver must know that AIDS is difficult to transmit, and he or she must communicate that knowledge by the ease in which he or she cares for the PWA. There is nothing more alienating for a hospitalized PWA and his family than having the minister enter the room unnecessarily covered from head to toe. The minister must know how to deal with the hospital staffperson who insists that the visitor follow complete isolation procedures. By the same token, the minister must be aware that on many occasions, isolation procedures are for the good of the patient, not the visitor. There-fore, the visitor must act in a way that will protect the PWA from any opportunistic diseases (such as the common cold) to which he or she may subject the patient. The minister must know when precautions are necessary and when they only add to the PWA's feeling of alienation.

If the pastoral counselor or caregiver discovers that he or she has great difficulty with homophobia, death, and contamination, it may be advisable that he or she make a referral to a minister who does not feel overly threatened by these pressures. It may make a difficult situation worse by treating the PWA like a leper, even if such behavior is not intentional (Dupree and Margo 1988, 2).

Lastly, the pastoral counselor or caregiver needs to have a strong sense of his or her own spirituality. Gay people with AIDS often have traveled much farther in their spiritual journey than their peers. This is due to the double pressure they feel from being a member of a sexual minority and from facing a life-threatening disease. Helpers, especially those from the religious community, need a mature and well-grounded spirituality if they want to provide authentic care to the PWA and FWA (Fortunato 1985, 119).

Grief and Loss

Historically, society has left the issues and concerns of death and dying to the church. With AIDS, however, the church oddly has abandoned that role. (Meyer 1986, 512).

The gay PWA, often a man in his twenties or thirties, may need to grieve the loss of his career, family, friends, hopes, sexuality, and dreams. The FWA's need to grieve is different from another family facing the death of a young adult. The FWA has to deal with the added issues of shame, alienation, secrecy, and guilt. Church people have, in the crisis of AIDS, the special opportunity to model the ministry of Jesus to Martha and Mary in a way that recent history has not offered (Quinn 1986, 505). Like Jesus, the pastoral counselor or caregiver must stand in the midst of suffering and dying and give testimony to the belief that life is stronger than death. AIDS may be the most difficult situation in which to do that, but it is also the situation in which this message is most needed.

Unfortunately, grief work with the gay PWA is further complicated by the homosexual issue. In chapter 8 of *Embracing the Exile: Healing Journeys for Gay Christians* (a book written to help psychotherapists and counselors make the work they do a more effective spiritual path), John E. Fortunato suggests that, from a psychotherapeutic point of view, being gay is in itself a grieving issue (Fortunato 1982, xv). Gay people must often "give up" many things, including the acceptance of their families and society; rearing their children if they have "come out" after being married and having children; many of their straight friends after they come out; being treated as equal by their straight friends and their coworkers; job security; legal and police protection; a secure place in religious institutions; freedom from the oppression that is often heaped upon minorities; and, if in a relationship, the legal, financial, and social benefits that accrue to married people (such as inheritance rights, going home for the holidays as a couple) (Fortunato 1982, 78–95). When dealing with the young man in this predicament, the pastoral counselor or caregiver must recognize that he or she is dealing with an additional layer of grief associated with being gay.

Grief is not reserved for the PWA or FWA whose son is close to death. The PWARC and the PHIV + are very susceptible to strong feelings of grief inasmuch as they often have to deal with the death of so many of their peers. One of the main reasons why many PWARC and PHIV + do not continue to attend support group meetings is that they attend the same group with PWA, and they cannot watch other young men and women deal with issues of death and dying. It is painful to see what is happening to their friends, and they find it extremely difficult, if not impossible, to see them without thinking, "In less than a year, that could be me!" Since the pastoral counselor is more apt to work with people at this early stage of the AIDS crisis, he or she must realize that grieving may be a powerful issue even if the client is years away from developing any symptoms.

Grief will almost always be an issue for the PWA, PWARC, and PHIV + whatever the case or at whatever stage of the disease. The PWA, PWARC, and PHIV + may need to deal with their bereavement with a representative of the church more than with any other service provider. For many persons there is something significantly different when a priest, deacon, sister, minister, or church representative works with or visits the gay PWA and his family. Something very powerful happens. Perhaps a representative of the church becomes a "God symbol," but, for whatever reason, something cathartic may begin to happen when a pastoral relationship is established. Although the catharsis does not always have to be positive (see the discussion of anger in chapter 2), it can be. When that happens the pastoral counselor or caregiver provides the PWA and the FWA with a connection to God that other professionals may be unable to duplicate. This God-connection is not meant to replace grief but rather to help the PWA and FWA gain some perspective on their grief and begin to see it in terms of their faith in a nonabandoning God of love.

The Spirituality of the
Gay Person with AIDS

When dealing with the gay PWA, it is particularly important for the pastoral counselor or caregiver to understand and be comfortable with the difference between spirituality and religion. Spirituality is a dimension of the human experience that transcends the immediate awareness of self. A person enters the realm of spirituality when questioning the meaning of life, when confronted with personal limitations, or when experiencing the unconditional love of another person. Spirituality is concerned with issues of meaning, hope, freedom, love, forgiveness, truth, and the image of God. Religion, on the other hand, is the ritualization or professionalization of these experiences. Religion is a human creation that tends to translate the spiritual experience into creed, cult, and community (Dunphy 1987, 1). Although religion and spirituality can exist in a delicate balance, there seems to be a primacy, inasmuch as religion exists to serve spirituality. This crucial distinction needs to be remembered when dealing with the gay PWA, precisely because he often presumes that because he is disconnected from organized religion he is also disconnected from his own personal spirituality, and subsequently alienated from God. This "disconnection" from organized religion can be due to factors such as: (1) dissatisfaction with a religious tradition (for example, the Roman Catholic teaching that he is "disordered," "unnatural," and "essentially self-indulgent"); (2) feelings of shame for being homosexual; and (3) a sense of guilt for homosexual activity.

One of the goals of pastoral counseling and care becomes helping the gay PWA understand the difference between spirituality and religion, helping him feel loved and accepted by God, and, if possible and appropriate, reconnecting him to his religious tradition or a more accepting religious tradition.

In attempting to reach this goal, the pastoral counselor or caregiver must recognize that there are some differences between the therapeutic and spiritual needs of the gay PWA. Fortunato discovered two important insights from his work with gay people. First, although the issues that brought gay people into counseling were basically the same as the issues of heterosexual people (such as death; serious illness; separation from or difficulties with a lover or spouse; the loss of a job; family problems; addiction; loneliness and hostility), these issues were more *intense* for the gay client (Fortunato 1982, 33). Fortunato attributes this intensity to a pervasive and unique form of rejection that only sexual minorities feel. Gay people may not have the opportunities to resolve the issues that bring people into counseling the way straight people resolve them (Fortunato 1982, 36). Consequently, he recommends a special sensitivity to gay people who come for therapeutic or spiritual guidance.

Sensitized by these issues, the pastoral counselor or caregiver can begin to address two powerful concerns: the gay PWA's anger and his need to discover the opportunity that is concealed in the disease.

Anger is a powerful source of stress in the life of a gay PWA. The flames of that anger can be fanned by feelings of alienation from the church and church representatives. It is understandable that a gay PWA might consider the pastoral counselor or caregiver to be a hypocrite, inasmuch as he or she represents an institution that declares its love and comfort for the sick (that is, the PWA), while often being indifferent, if not hostile, to the gay person before the illness puts the PWA in the hospital (an example of being put in the double bind). It should not surprise the minister that the gay PWA may, at first, treat him or her with distance, indifference, suspicion, and often anger. These possible reactions demand that the pastoral counselor or caregiver be given some special preparation. He or she will require an extra measure of commitment, patience, loyalty, and perseverance, as well as a tremendous amount of time, if he or she chooses to do ministry to PWAs and their families (Shelp & Sunderland 1987, 100).

On the question of acceptance of one's sexuality, the pastoral counselor or caregiver may be able to help the gay PWA acknowledge his sexual orientation as a part of God's creation. If the gay PWA's God is a God who inspires fear, then anger over his homosexuality might better be left alone. However, if the gay PWA can work through his anger at a God who punishes and comes to believe in a God of love, then sexuality, both homosexuality and heterosexuality, can be accepted as a gift from God that, like all other gifts, can be treasured.

Now you, like most gay people I know, had to reject the Church and society's definition of who God is in order to accept yourself as God made you to be. Through this painful metamorphosis comes the realization that the homosexual condition, like the heterosexual condition, is a gift from God, and if only we could accept that basic fact, so much pain would be obliterated. Everyone who cares to know, knows that people have as much freedom in the choice of their sexual orientation as they do in the color of their eyes. There is no reputable psychiatrist or psychologist that would postulate otherwise (Lynch 1987, 15).

Once the gay PWA is beyond anger, the minister can begin to guide the person into understanding that there is a gift in the midst of the suffering. For those who are able to see it, the suffering of AIDS can be understood as sharing in the suffering of Christ. They come to realize that there is some value to suffering and understand the place of suffering in God's scheme of things. These people, more than most, comprehend Paul's meaning when he wrote: "In my own flesh I fill up what is lacking in the sufferings of Christ for the sake of his body, the church" (Col. 1:24, New American Bible).

The PWA, pushed to the edge of his life at an early age, can experience great joy from God's creation that he took for granted up until now. Friends and family, nature, spirituality, and the arts, take on a new meaning. The PWA can attain a wisdom far beyond his years. He learns to live each day to its fullest, not simply because his number of days has been cut short, but also because he has discovered a new respect for life in the present. He can be less distracted by building a career, amassing wealth, or planning for the distant future. Living life in the present can give him insights that few of us take time to appreciate. The PWA can reverse the role and begin to minister to the pastoral counselor or caregiver out of the wealth of his experience. Those who offer to care for the PWA and the FWA should be ready to receive as much as, if not more than, they give (Stulz 1986, 510).

The gay PWA should be encouraged to believe that he is a gift to those around him, the pastoral counselor or caregiver included. As Christians we have an obligation to care for "the poor," so when we have an opportunity to do that, we should be grateful.

A simple story may help in comprehending this idea:

An American traveled to India to visit an old friend who was doing missionary work in that country. While the two of them were walking through the streets of Calcutta a beggar approached the visitor and asked for alms. Instinctively, the American reached into his pocket and placed some change in the old man's hand, at which point the missionary instructed his American friend to say "thank you" to the beggar. Not wanting to make an issue out of the experience, the American never questioned his friend about what happened until the day he was departing. "Remember the day I gave some change to the old man in Calcutta?" "Yes," the missionary replied. "Well, why did you tell me to thank him? Didn't you really mean that he should thank me?" In a voice that indicated that he expected the question, the missionary gently answered: "No, because in this country we believe that the poor give us the opportunity to perform a good deed for which there is far greater reward. And so, we thank them for the chance to put our faith into practice."

Doctors, nurses, social workers, family members, friends, and church people *need* the PWA just as much as the PWA needs them. This mystery may be difficult for the PWA to understand. Yet through the mutuality of the pastoral counselor or caregiver, the PWA may come to see this more clearly.

John Fortunato tells a story from his youth. He went to a young priest and confessed that he was gay. The priest told him that God loved him *anyway*. What the priest really told him was that being gay was sinful, but God was able to overlook this fault. Fortunato describes the experience as a "strange liberation" (Fortunato 1982, 12). Let us hope that the crisis of AIDS has raised the issue of homosexuality in such a way that it will help the pastoral counselor or caregiver to delete the "anyway" as he or she reassures the PWA of God's love.

Suicide

The pastoral counselor or caregiver must develop a special sensitivity to the issue of suicide for the sake of the patient, the family, and his or her own emotional health.

It would be laudable if every PWA had the kind of spirituality that would allow him to understand the importance of offering his life to God as Jesus did in the Garden of Gethsemane (Luke 22:42). However, the average PWA, PWARC, or PHIV+ may not be able to reach such heights of spirituality, and the effects of the disease on the central nervous systems may rob him of the opportunity. In any case, the pastoral counselor must try to understand the despair that must be part of the everyday life of a PWA, PWARC, or PHIV+.

The weight of this disease and the constellation of psychosocial stressors (such as guilt, low self-esteem, shame, alienation, fear, stigma, discrimination; see chapter 2) that surround it may drive the PWA, PWARC, or PHIV+ to consider taking his own life. On the physical level, the PWA is subject to debilitating weakness, wasting, constant fever, nagging diarrhea, the potential loss of mobility, the prospect of around-the-clock care, and vulnerability to any number of opportunistic diseases that can take his sense of touch, taste, sight, and mind. It is difficult to think of another disease that is so merciless and debilitating. It is no wonder that thoughts of suicide are on the mind of everyone afflicted with this disease. The best suicide prevention might be giving the patient the space to vent feelings of despair to lessen the likelihood of unexpressed feeling welling up and overtaking him in a moment of crisis.

By the same token, the pastoral counselor or caregiver, possibly more than any other counseling professional, can offer the gift of acceptance to the family of the PWA, PWARC, or PHIV+ who does take his life. As a representative of the faith community, the pastoral counselor or caregiver will not only remind the family that it is not our job to judge but to help them through the doubly difficult grieving process that must follow losing a loved one to AIDS and suicide.

Lastly, the pastoral counselor or caregiver must come to grips with his or her own feelings about suicide. Just as we would counsel a doctor or nurse not to see the PWA's death as a medical failure, so the pastoral counselor or caregiver cannot interpret his or her relationship with a PWA as a failure if the PWA should commit suicide. It may be of some consolation to know that many moral theologians would be hard-pressed to find "full consent of the will" in any person suffering from a medical, social, and psychological crisis as profound as AIDS.

The Worried Well

People with full-fledged AIDS are not the only ones who suffer from the psychosocial stresses of AIDS. The PWARC and PHIV+ feel many of these stresses and some that are endemic to their condition. Although the PWARC is somewhat debilitated, he is not seriously sick or in imminent danger. The PHIV+, although he will be infected all his life, is, by nature of the definition of his condition, without symptoms. However, both groups of people live in fear and wonder if or when they will develop the symptoms that will result in a diagnosis of AIDS. The pressure and worry that are a part of their everyday lives lead some to say, "I would almost rather get AIDS. That way, I would at least know and could plan my life. The uncertainty is terrible" (Stulz 1986, 511).

AIDS also takes a terrible toll on gay men in general. Because of their sexual history or just because they may have so many friends who are HIV+ or who have been diagnosed with ARC or AIDS, many gay men live with the constant worry that "I will be next." The pastoral counselor or caregiver must be aware of their plight because they, just as the people who are already sick, may need special attention. Like their PWA, PWARC, and PHIV+ peers, they are subject to many of the same feelings: fear, anger, the need for secrecy, denial, and confusion, to name a few. It should come as no surprise to the pastoral counselor or caregiver that, after caring for a PWA, he or she may receive a request for an appointment from one of that PWA's gay friends. These people often live in mortal fear of each new piece of information about the incubation time for the virus. Unlike any other group of people their age, gay men must face the prospect of their own premature death. Therefore, a service provider like the pastoral counselor or caregiver must be careful not to write off the PWARC's or PHIV+'s reactions as hysterical.

The minister should realize that AIDS is a disease that affects the entire gay community, including those who, at least so far, have not gotten it. Gay men may have anywhere from one to dozens of friends who are into the throes of the disease. They must experience the kind of grieving that senior citizens feel as they watch their peers die off. The only differences are that young gay men do not have the wisdom that often comes with old age nor the satisfaction of having lived a full life.

Because of the AIDS connection with the homosexual, AIDS has also contributed to homophobia. AIDS has exacerbated discrimination against publicly gay people by employers, insurance companies, health care providers, churches, housing authorities, and the government. AIDS has pushed many young gay men back into the closet and prevented others from coming to grips with their membership in a sexual minority. AIDS has had a profound effect on almost every part of the homosexual community.

The crisis of AIDS spills on those affected with the disease as well as those who are associated with the disease. AIDS is no longer just a concern for the PWA, PWARC, PHIV + and the FWA; it is a societal issue. The pastoral counselor or caregiver needs to recognize the breadth and the depth of this tragedy in order to face it in the best way possible.

Chapter 2

THE EMOTIONAL
STRESSES OF AIDS

Loss and grief are facts of life for every family, but especially for a family affected by a disease as devastating as AIDS. The loss of any family member creates a family crisis, but this is especially so when a young family member's death comes as a radical interruption of the life cycle. The helping professional needs to understand the AIDS experience in order to provide effective treatment, pastoral counseling, or pastoral care. This chapter will assist the helper in understanding the emotional stressors that AIDS brings to a person and family such as loss, anger, fear, and guilt. An awareness of the breadth and depth of the grieving process in the family with AIDS can help the caregiver assist the family in recovering as fully as possible.

Researchers project that in the 1990s, every extended American family will have a member infected with the Human Immunodeficiency Virus (HIV). This forecast is based on statistics presented in the summer of 1988 at the Fourth International Conference on AIDS held in Stockholm, which predicted that by 1992 there will be 365,000 to 380,000 cases of AIDS in the United States. People in the field extrapolate that for every person with AIDS (PWA) there are ten people with AIDS Related Complex (ARC), and fifty people who test HIV+. If this equation holds true, then by 1992 there will be an additional 3,650,000 people who have ARC and 18,250,000 who test sereo-positive. Thus, AIDS and the psychosocial stressors that accompany it will reach epidemic proportions for the American family. AIDS could become a national bereavement issue. The family, along with the nation, needs to understand what we are up against in this epidemic.

Families who must deal with the threat of a gay son's death to AIDS, or his actual death, have a unique opportunity to change. The diagnosis of AIDS, ARC, or HIV + may present the family with an occasion for working out an unresolved family issue that might never have been confronted without a crisis. The pastoral counselor or caregiver, because of his or her connection to the family and the rituals that often revolve around the serious illness or death of a family member, has an unequaled opportunity to facilitate this process (Friedman 1985, 169–70).

When dealing with grief-laden situations like AIDS, it is important for the helping professional to (1) know the total family configuration; (2) be aware of the functioning position of the gay PWA in the family; (3) be able to appraise the overall level of life adaptation in the family; (4) have his or her own emotional life under reasonable control without the interference of denial; and (5) respect the denial that operates in the FWA (Bowen 1978, 328–29).

The family with AIDS (FWA) will face many issues of bereavement and will take many steps on their way to acceptance of this illness and preparation for death. There will be an initial crisis after the diagnosis that may be marked by intense grief or denial and false optimism. Then there will be a transitional phase in which the PWA, PWARC, PHIV +, or FWA may experience a wide range of emotions (Walker 1987b, 2). The most frequently encountered emotions will be considered in this chapter as some of the psychosocial stressors that affect persons and families with AIDS. With therapeutic intervention by a knowledgeable professional, the FWA may be able to attain a level of acceptance that allows them to face as many of the stressors as possible and, when they have reached their limit, to defend themselves with a healthy level of denial.

Loss

One of the most powerful psychosocial stressors for those affected by AIDS is the issue of loss. Although many people equate loss with death, death is not the only loss. Daily life is filled with "little deaths." Loss then is any event or action that takes from us something we have had and valued. Loss leaves a trail of grief in its wake. Because loss is a matter of having and then not having, it is markedly different than deprivation, which is never having in the first place. Loss is to deprivation as going blind is to being blind from birth. Therefore, loss can be moved out of the realm of the medical model, which sees it as failure, and into the realm of the health model, where loss becomes a part of the "normal."

Loss can be divided into some major categories. Under the label of "predictable" losses we find: (1) loss of a significant person (through death, aging, divorce); (2) loss of a part or function of the self (amputation, impotence, blindness, baldness); (3) loss of material objects; (4) loss of trust, freedom, love, youth, security, hope; and (5) developmental loss (weaning, starting school, leaving home). Less predictable losses that impact the family include: (1) divorce; (2) death, particularly accidental or by murder or suicide; (3) victimization (rape, assault, hijacking, disappearance, or kidnapping); (4) natural and man-made disasters.

The PWA, PWARC, PHIV +, or the FWA can feel loss in at least the following ways:

1. *The loss of sexuality.* Now infected with the HIV virus the PWA knows that he will be contagious for the rest of his life. Even if a vaccine for AIDS is developed, those who are seropositive will probably remain that way for the rest of their lives. This results in an attitude about sexuality that one PWA chooses to call the "poison dart syndrome."

2. *The loss of romance.* Unless a PWA, PWARC, or PHIV + is in a relationship or begins to date another person, he may feel as though he has no romantic future. Confiding his medical status to another person can be the beginning of the end of any future relationship. "We can still be friends" is the response that many persons affected by the AIDS virus dread hearing. When questioned as to why he had eaten almost every meal out at a restaurant, a PWA responded that going out to eat with friends was the only romantic thing left in his life.

3. *Loss of control over life.*   The PWA, PWARC, or PHIV+ often feels a general sense of loss over his body and his life. This can be exacerbated by the medical model that may lack an effective treatment plan due to the lack of knowledge about the disease. These feelings are particularly relevant to the counselor since counseling seeks to help the client gain a sense of control over his or her life. It may be fair to conclude that many, if not most, PWAs, PWARCs, and PHIV+s would benefit from a counseling relationship.

4. *Loss of identity.*   Many people in their twenties, thirties, and forties identify themselves by what they do for a living. A successful career is perhaps one of the most important parts of a person's self-image. The diagnosis of AIDS almost always means the end of work, and the diagnosis of ARC, depending on the route the disease takes, can mean the same thing. Therefore, young gay PWAs and PWARCs, many of whom are well educated and upwardly mobile, must often terminate their jobs and careers decades before they are prepared to (Walker 1988, 26).

5. *Loss of a lover.*   Oftentimes the PWA, PWARC, or PHIV+ may have lost a lover to the disease, or, in some cases, to suicide. The bereaved must often bury his loss under the cloud of shame, guilt, secrecy, and stigma. He must also grieve the fact that he may have been left at risk of the disease (Gilbert 1988, 42). If the PWA, PWARC, or PHIV+ is in a relationship with someone who is not sero-positive, he may have to grieve the loss of his partner who may choose to leave him rather than risk infection.

6. *Loss of support.*   If he has lost his lover to AIDS, the PWA, PWARC, or PHIV+ must do much of his grieving without the common social supports available to other people. AIDS often strips away the support the grieving people and families can receive from neighbors, church, coworkers, and other family members. If a family cannot tell people about what is wrong with their son, brother, or lover, then how can they accept support from people who, often with good intentions, ask questions about the diagnosis, prognosis, or cause of death? In many ways, AIDS cuts people off from the support that they could find in everyday relationships.

7. *The loss of meaning and hope.*   Like all of us, PWAs need meaning and hope in their lives as they struggle to cope with the

tragic toll that AIDS will take on their lives. Like all of us, gay men give meaning and hope to their lives by creating a sense of identity and self-worth. This is often accomplished through sources of self-worth such as personal and professional relationships; the acceptance and respect received from these relationships; personal and material satisfaction received from working; participation in organized religion; and from an experience of God. The gay PWA may feel that many, if not most, of these elements are threatened or lost due to his diagnosis.

The sense of loss in the PWA, PWARC, PHIV +, FWA, and the entire gay community can be overwhelming. The gay community may feel that the liberties that have come to them so late and after such a difficult struggle are now lost due to the AIDS crisis and its unfortunate preeminence within the homosexual community.

Anger

Anger is everywhere in the lives of those affected by AIDS.

The PWA, PWARC, or PHIV + often feels a generalized anger at life. It is common to hear him rage: "There is no justice in this world." "There are lots of people worse than me, why did this have to happen to me?" and, "All I wanted to do was love someone." If the PWA's spirituality is founded on a connection that God is controlling and judgmental, he will often be angry at God for "punishing" him with AIDS. The PWA may be angry at his lover for infecting him; for not being infected; for the possibility that the lover may leave, especially if the lover is not infected; or angry for fear that, if he tells his lover how he really feels, the lover may abandon him. The PWA may be furious at a health care system that does not have answers to his questions, is still experimenting with treatment at his peril, and is so expensive. Often, people in this situation are irate with the state and federal bureaucracy for the delays in funding research and the paucity of financial assistance given to PWAs and to those who work with them. Lastly, the feeling of loss can contribute to an already powerful sense of anger, making it almost overwhelming.

The FWA can be angry at the PWA, PWARC, or PHIV+ because of his alleged irresponsibility or sinfulness that has brought shame upon the family. A family that discovers the homosexual orientation of a son through the announcement of AIDS, ARC, or HIV+ faces a terrible double shock that can elicit even more anger (see "The Double Barrel Effect" in chapter 3). Because so many PWAs return to their family of origin as the disease progresses, mothers, fathers, sisters, and brothers can become very angry at having to assume responsibility for the financial needs of the PWA not to mention the physical burdens of caring for a terminally ill person.

The PWA's lover may have a different set of angry feelings. He may begin to question his lover's fidelity, especially if they have been together for a number of years, and he may assume that his lover became sero-positive while they were together. No matter when the PWA was exposed to virus, the PWA's partner may be angry because he feels that the man that he is in love with has threatened his life. The lover may have unexpressed feelings of anger because he cannot discuss other important issues with his PWA lover for fear that such discussions may add to the stress the PWA is already experiencing.

This process can develop into a cycle of anger in which the inability to express anger makes a person more angry and, in turn, more unwilling to express it. If the PWA begins to depend more and more on his family of origin and that family of origin is unaccepting of the PWA's lover, then the lover may be painted out of the picture at a time when the PWA needs him the most and at a time when he may need the PWA the most. This lack of acceptance at such a critical time results in anger and hurt on the part of the lover.

Lastly, young people in relationships do not expect to have to deal with chronic illness, debilitating disease, and premature death. Those issues are "reserved" for the elderly. A PWA's lover may feel cheated by what is happening to his mate and himself, especially if the burden of care—whether financial, physical, or emotional—falls on him. Robbed of his plans, dreams, and hopes for this relationship, the PWA's lover may experience an enormous amount of resentment and anger for what is happening to him. If they are a very private couple, the situation at home may be unknown to the lover's family and coworkers. Therefore, the PWA's lover may have to take shelter in lies and excuses to explain his frequent absences and exhaustion not to mention the fact that his family and coworkers will not be available to support him during the crisis of his lover's illness and death. Under these circumstances it would be hard not to project feelings of anger onto his PWA lover (Shelp & Sunderland 1987, 47).

No matter where the anger comes from, who is expressing it and where it may be directed, it is important that the PWA, PWARC, PHIV +, and his family learn to express their anger. Unexpressed anger may, at the private end of the spectrum, become depression or, at the public end of the spectrum, develop into rage (Woititz 1985, 36).

Fear

If fear is not the most potent psychosocial stressor, then it is certainly the most present; it seems to appear everywhere and affect everyone.

The gay PWA, PWARC, or PHIV + lives in dread of losing his lover while the lover fears for the health of the PWA as well as his own health. The PWA, PWARC, or PHIV +, along with his lover, has a fear of who is responsible for this infection. Or to put it bluntly in the words of a PWA, "Did I kill you, or did you kill me?"

The PWA, PWARC, or PHIV +, along with his family and lover, often fears that AIDS is a punishment from God for being gay or sexually active. If he has that kind of image of God, then he may face death with an overwhelming sense of guilt and apprehension.

One of these real fears is that the patient will be denied religious understanding and compassion—that the patient by virtue of past (or current) behavior is no longer eligible for the care and concern of the church, synagogue, or religious tradition from which he or she speaks. Taking this even further, many patients deduce that they are not eligible for the care and concern of God. They feel ultimately rejected and abandoned, cast out (Marshall 1987, 18).

Everyone affected by AIDS fears the disease. What route will it take? What symptoms will I have? How long will it last? Will there be much pain? Will I lose my mind to dementia?

Guilt

Guilt can be a feeling of wrongdoing, a sense of wickedness, and a perception of oneself as "not good" (Woititz 1985, 39). If the PWA, PWARC, or PHIV+ internalizes any of the negative messages that society sends him, he may begin to believe that AIDS is a punishment from God, that he is intrinsically evil, and that he deserves to suffer and does not merit medical care. It is not hard to imagine how a guilt-ridden PWA, PWARC, or PHIV+ might accept the "blame the victim" stance, a phenomenon that often occurs when morality becomes interwoven with disease. Subsequently, the patient may stop taking his medication or cancel his doctor appointments; he may refuse the opportunity for therapy, pastoral care, or pastoral counseling and begin to distance himself from friends, family, and lover; and he may seriously consider suicide.

If the PWA, PWARC, or PHIV+ was in a relationship with a PWA who died, he may experience "survivor guilt." Questions like "Why did he die and I'm still alive?" can begin to haunt the surviving lover.

The FWA is not immune to guilt. Parents of a gay man, especially fathers, may feel that they failed in raising their son. They conclude that they must have done something wrong or else their child would have been heterosexual. If they knew that their son was gay and reacted negatively to his sexual orientation (more than 50 percent of all families do), they may feel guilty for not having accepted him as he is. If their lack of acceptance contributed to the gay son's "leaving town" (see "The Emotional Cut-Off" in chapter 4), and they think he was infected with AIDS in the "big city," then they are apt to feel even more responsible. If, however, they were not aware of their son's sexual orientation until his diagnosis, then they may feel he never trusted them enough to tell them about his life-style. Parents in this situation might feel that they failed because their son could not confide in his mother or father. The FWA may refuse to take their son home to die because they fear family, friends, and neighbors would learn the truth about their son and brother. This all too common scenario can generate feelings of rejection, neglect, and abandonment in the PWA and feelings of guilt in the FWA.

In August 1984, Barbara Peabody, author of *The Screaming Room,* and two other mothers founded Mothers for AIDS Patients (MAP). Realizing that AIDS is a terribly lonely disease for the mother as well as the patient, they created an organization to offer the members services as "substitute mothers" for rejected AIDS patients (Peabody 1986, 254).

Unfortunately, the parent who is accepting of his or her son's sexual orientation and dedicated to his health is not exempt from feelings of guilt, even if they are only "perceived" feelings of guilt. Often parents feel a need to save their children from illness, sorrow, failure, and death. This is difficult to accomplish under any circumstance but especially in the case of AIDS. In case of a parent who is not accepting of his or her son's sexual orientation, there could be a sense of guilt over that parent's failure to save his or her son from homosexuality and from a homosexual life-style.

Like people who lose a loved one to suicide, war, or murder, the FWA may experience what has been termed the "survivor-victim" syndrome. This phrase describes the unresolved grief and guilt that is left behind in the wake of a tragedy like AIDS. Parents in this situation may begin to compensate for their guilt by reacting in an inappropriate way toward another child.

Guilt, like anger, is a many-headed dragon for the FWA.

Shame and Stigma

Shame, a feeling closely linked to guilt, is a sense of inadequacy, worthlessness, and an image that "I am no good." Overcoming these feelings can often be a life-long struggle (Woititz 1985, 3). It may be even more difficult for a person who is threatened by a disease like AIDS.

Shame is generated by a variety of factors, but one of the major contributors to shame is the mode of contagion of the disease. The most common way that AIDS is transmitted in the homosexual community is through sexual contact. The venereal nature of its transmission makes AIDS a magnet for shame and the subsequent stigma.

> Venereal germs became a special category of disease agents which were viewed as willfully contracted. If VD could no longer be considered a manifestation of moral corruption because its microbial cause was visible, then it could become an even worse disorder because its route of transmission was an act chosen in violation of social mores and religious laws. Of all the diseases which served simultaneously as symptoms of evil and as punishment in themselves, VD retained both qualities in the U.S. culture (Patton 1985, 59).

Sexually transmitted diseases elicit strong reactions, often including condemnation, alienation, and judgment. Probably more than any other person in contemporary society, the PWA, PWARC, PHIV +, and his family are likely to feel the shame and stigma that the diagnosis of sero-positivity will bring on their heads. Because AIDS is often perceived as a gay man's disease, this shame and stigma are often increased.

Instead of looking at the broader issues and how society has "set up" the gay community to carry this disease for the rest of us, people are much more apt to look for a moral scapegoat. They have found their scapegoat in the gay man, and they project stigma and shame on him and his family.

The shame that the gay PWA, PWARC, or PHIV + can feel on the inside is often externalized, resulting in an overwhelming feeling of stigmatization (Walker 1988, 29). AIDS presents a double invitation to stigmatize: not only is AIDS associated with issues that society dreads and rejects (sexual deviation, death, and sexually transmitted diseases), but some of the symptoms of the disease (such as Kaposi's Sarcoma, wasting, and physical dependency) can be so obvious that they thrust the PWA into the public forum where he is subjected to the rejection of society.

AIDS, with all its psychosocial stressors, its ability to generate homophobic reactions, and the sexual manner of its transmission, provides a perfect opportunity for the breeding of shame and stigma. Precisely when the PWA, PWARC, or PHIV + seeks support and a sense of belonging, he frequently meets the progeny of shame and stigma: prejudice, discrimination, condemnation, and abandonment. What he needs is an atmosphere of acceptance and love that can facilitate physical, emotional, and spiritual health. What he gets is often very different.

Secrecy

The shame and stigma of AIDS often results in a reaction of secrecy. PWAs, PWARCs, PHIV + s, and their families keep their diagnosis secret in order to protect themselves from the negative reactions of family, friends, neighbors, church, and society. In an attempt to protect themselves from rejection, they also cut themselves off from a variety of support sources. This adds to the feelings of shame and stigma, creating a vicious circle.

Secrecy can be omnipresent in the AIDS system. The gay PWA, PWARC, or PHIV + may choose not to tell his family of his diagnosis in the same way he chooses not to tell them of his sexual orientation. He may tell only a few friends, for fear they will start to treat him differently or, in some cases, gradually abandon him. He may avoid telling his employer for fear of losing his job and having his coworkers refuse to work with him, thereby forcing his employer to let him go. After divulging their secret to employers or coworkers, many PWAs and PWARCs are given leaves of absence with pay, or their services are donated to AIDS organizations so that the employee has a job and the employer can soothe his or her conscience for wanting to get rid of a potential problem.

The need for secrecy is so powerful in such people's lives that sometimes the PWA, PWARC, or PHIV + refuses to tell his lover of the diagnosis. The Ackerman Institute has noted that some of its clients who want couples therapy request that their lovers not be told about the diagnosis. Although this is an extreme example of how the right to confidentiality of one client can clash with the right to know of another client, it does show how much some people want to protect their privacy when it comes to AIDS (Walker 1987a, 7).

The PWARC is especially tempted to maintain secrecy in the workplace because, although he may be in generally good health, his energy level is usually compromised. He may need to find a variety of excuses to explain his exhaustion, irritability, and poor performance. Not knowing how long he may stay in the ARC stage, he will want to protect his position for as long as possible. All of these factors add up to a serious need for secrecy in the life of a PWARC.

Because of their fear of the unknown, the FWA may choose to hide their son's diagnosis from most, if not all, parts of their lives: neighbors, friends, church, employers, and coworkers.

Although secrecy is understandable under such circumstances, it unfortunately adds to the already high level of stress that surrounds a person with AIDS.

The Life-Threatening Nature of AIDS

The PWA, PWARC, and PHIV+ resent and resist being labeled "terminal." Although they are more than willing to recognize that AIDS is a life-threatening disease, they do not want to think of themselves, nor do they want other people to think of them, as people who are dying of AIDS. Rather, they are people who are living with AIDS. A terminal diagnosis can add to the depression and fatalism that are already too much a part of the disease. Trying to live with AIDS is the only chance these people have, a chance that is constantly being improved as scientists continue to discover ways to ward off the infectious diseases that are so often the cause of death.

Labeling this crisis a "life-threatening" disease rather than a "terminal" disease does not, unfortunately, relieve the PWA, PWARC, or PHIV+ from having to deal with the issues of loss that this illness raises. (See the discussion of "Loss" earlier in this chapter.)

Disruption of the Family Life Cycle

Many of the emotional stressors already discussed contribute to the disruption of the life plans of the PWA, PWARC, or PHIV+ and his family. Family system therapists are particularly sensitive to the patterns found in families as they move through time. This pattern is referred to as the "life cycle," that is, "a series of stages or 'categories' which occur in a sequential order of approximately similar sequence from one family to another" (Paolino 1978, 338).

> The family life cycle perspective views symptoms and dysfunction in relation to normal function over time. It frames problems within the course the family has moved along in its past, the tasks that it is presently trying to master and the future towards which it is moving (Walsh 1982, 167).

A quick survey of the accompanying chart of the family life cycle reveals that many categories of this life cycle are significantly different for the gay man while some of them are completely denied him when he suffers from AIDS. The most glaring difference is the time of life at which a person needs to deal with the loss of a lover and other peers, as well as the preparation for one's own death. What "should" and normally does happen to a family member in his or her seventies or eighties happens to the gay PWA in his thirties or forties, and as the disease spreads, in his twenties. The death of a young adult assaults the family life cycle and can send shock waves through the entire multigenerational family system. The threat of death carried by AIDS disrupts the life plans of both the PWA and the FWA. The PWA must come to grips with the enormous sense of loss as he sees his dreams for the future fade away. The FWA, especially the parents, must deal with issues that they are not supposed to have to deal with: the health and welfare of their adult child, the loss of security that an adult child represents to their old age, and the death and burial of one of their offspring. Parents often respond, "It isn't supposed to be this way!" The grief of such a life cycle tragedy can be exacerbated if, as the PWA approaches death, the family chooses to keep their son's illness or the cause of his illness a secret. This can cut the family off from the normal support of family, friends, neighbors, coworkers, church, and others (Shelp and Sunderland 1987, 46). Of course, telling other people can also cut the FWA off from the same normal support systems.

FAMILY LIFE CYCLE

Stages	Emotional Process of Transition
Between families: the unattached young	Accepting parent-offspring separation
The joining of families through marriage: the newly married couple	Commitment to new system
The family with young children	Accepting new generation of members into the system
The family with adolescents	Increasing flexibility of family boundaries to include children's independence
Launching children and moving on	Accepting a multitude of exits from and entries into family
The family in later life	Accepting the shifting of later generational roles

(Walsh 1982, 176)

Second Order Changes

(a) Differentiation of self in relation to family of origin
(b) Development of intimate peer relationships
(c) Establishment of self in work

(a) Formation of marital system
(b) Realignment of relationship with extended families and
     friends to include spouse

(a) Adjusting to marital system to make space for child(ren)
(b) Taking on parenting roles
(c) Realignment of relationship with extended family to
     include parenting and grandparenting roles

(a) Shifting of parent-child relationships to permit adolescents
     to move in and out of the system
(b) refocus on midlife and career issues
(c) Beginning shift toward concerns for older generation

(a) Renegotiation of marital system as a dyad
(b) Development of adult-to-adult relationships between
     grown children and their parents
(c) Realignment of relationships to include in-laws and
     grandchildren
(d) Dealing with disabilities and death of parents and
     grandparents

(a) Maintaining own or couple functioning and interests in
     face of physiological decline; exploration of new familial
     and social role options
(b) Support for more central role for middle generation
(c) Making room in the system for the wisdom and
     experiences of the elderly; supporting the older
     generation without overfunctioning for them
(d) Dealing with loss of spouse, siblings and other peers, and
     preparing for own death; life review and integration

Chapter 3

A SYSTEM OF PSYCHOSOCIAL STRESSORS

In addition to the emotional factors considered in the previous chapter, there are a number of additional factors that add stress to the situation of all of those living with AIDS. In the AIDS crisis all of these factors are interrelated in a "system" of psychosocial stressors that weighs upon the person with AIDS (PWA), person with AIDS Related Complex (PWARC), person with Human Immunodeficiency Virus, (PHIV+), and family with AIDS (FWA). In order to understand the magnitude of the problem, we need to move away from "linear" causation (that is, the "billard ball" effect, in which A causes B, B causes C, C causes D, etc.; each having its own discrete identity or input resulting in E [Fig. 1]) and "multiple" causation (the theory that a group of factors [A, B, C, D] when pulled together will produce E [Fig. 2]), to "systems" causation (Fig. 3), an understanding that sees each factor, including the end result operating as part of the whole (Friedman 1985, 16).

According to this understanding we are looking at a complex interrelated and stress-provoking circle of psychosocial factors (Fig. 4). This chapter will review the complexity of a number of these interrelated factors to provide a broader understanding of the crisis that AIDS represents to families.

Homophobia

Because of AIDS' connection with homosexuals, there is the multifaceted issue of homophobia, in addition to the fear felt by

Linear Causation (Figure 1):

A $\longrightarrow$ B $\longrightarrow$ C $\longrightarrow$ D = E

Multiple Causation (Figure 2):

A   B   C   D

E

Systems Causation (Figure 3):

Circle of Psychosocial Factors (Figure 4):

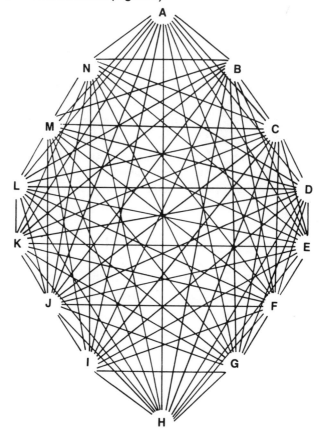

the PWA that was discussed in the previous chapter. John Patten, a family systems therapist on the AIDS Project at the Ackerman Institute in New York City, divides this fear into three categories: homophobia, homo-negativism, and homo-confusion. Homophobia is "the total rejection of homosexuality as a normal and acceptable human choice about one's sexual preference." Homophobia, he claims, can be very subtle and present even among professionals who presumably attempt to help their gay clients. One of the most powerful symptoms of homophobia is the tendency to blame gay men for the AIDS epidemic.

> Gay men are often scapegoated in AIDS prevention programs. The assumption is that if it had not been for gay men and their sexual practices, AIDS would not be a problem. Thus control of homosexuality, rather than the disease, becomes the solution (Frutchey 1988, 3).

Patten defines homo-negativism as a more common, although less outright, attitude that does not lead people to actively discriminate against or condemn homosexuals, but prevents them from truly accepting someone in the family who is involved in a gay relationship. Homo-negativism might sound like this: "I don't care what my son does in the privacy of his own bedroom as long as he doesn't expect to bring his lover home for Thanksgiving dinner." Lastly, Patten proposes that the largest group includes those who do not have any strongly held views but are confused by all the conflicting information they get from the media and other sources. He calls these people the homo-confused (Patten 1988, 37).

Homophobia, the most virulent form of homosexual fear, seems to spill over into a variety of places and persons. The medical profession is seriously affected by homophobia. Extensive education does not seem to provide an antidote for this form of prejudice (Frutchey 1988, 3). The gay person can suffer from a form of this called "internalized homophobia," a symptom that the person has not completely accepted himself.

> In the face of a catastrophic illness like AIDS, latent homophobia, even in a previously well-adjusted gay man, can reassert itself and

take the form of accepting society's negative judgments about gay men who have AIDS: for example, "Maybe God is punishing me for my lifestyle" (Dunphy 1987, 2).

This feeling can be aggravated by fear of AIDS contamination and a belief that the illness is God's punishment for the gay PWA's sexual orientation and life-style. Internalized homophobia can produce self-hatred, alienation from one's self and others, lowered self-esteem, the fear of external judgment, and depression (Walker 1987a, 6).

AIDS Hysteria, the "Other" Epidemic

Fear of AIDS can become so excessive and unmanageable that it can mushroom into hysteria, an unreasonable, irrational, and exaggerated fear. This may be due to the fact that AIDS is contagious but also because it is often a sexually transmitted disease.

For the past 150 years, people who suffer from infectious diseases have also been the victims of negative religious and moral attitudes. Cholera, an epidemic that struck the United States in 1832, 1849, and 1866, is a devastating disease characterized by diarrhea, acute spasmodic vomiting, painful cramps, consequent dehydration, cyanosis, and possibly death within hours or days following the onset of symptoms. The cholera virus is easily spread by any pathway (such as food, water, hands) to the digestive tract. During the epidemic of 1832, cholera was considered the scourge of the sinful, an inescapable judgment of God upon people who violated the laws of God. It was thought that only dirty, intemperate people were at risk and that the "respectable" were immune. Although the disease or vice connection still persisted during the 1849 cholera epidemic, the needs of those orphaned and made destitute were finally addressed by "Christian gentlemen." During the last attack of cholera in 1866, advances in medical understanding of the disease moved society from condemning the disease to controlling it by means of personal hygiene, sanitation, disinfection, and quarantine.

The relationship between religious values and society's response to infectious disease has not been restricted to cholera.

In the last hundred years people have applied the same attitudes that they once applied to cholera to venereal disease, namely, that sexually transmitted diseases are a punishment from God on sinful, "dirty" people. (See discussion of shame in chapter 2.) The discovery of a cure for syphilis and gonorrhea in 1932 gave society a brief respite from its need to scapegoat and condemn. However, with the onslaught of AIDS in the early 1980s, people have a new identified patient to project their fears on. This simplistic, irrational overreaction takes many forms.

Some think that research and treatment is a waste of money because they believe AIDS will be eliminated when homosexuals are eliminated—the purpose of the disease in the first place. In the words of Ronald S. Goodwin, then executive member of the Moral Majority, "What I see is a commitment to spend our tax dollars on research to allow these diseased homosexuals to go back to their perverted practices without any standard of accountability" (Shelp & Sunderland 1987, 19).

Patrick Buchanan, conservative columnist and former White House Director of Communications, wrote in 1985 that the "essence" of homosexual life is "runaway promiscuity," which leads to illness and death. "Call it nature's retribution, God's will, the wages of sin, paying the piper, ecological kickback, whatever phraseology you prefer" (Shelp & Sunderland, 21). While William F. Buckley, Jr., proposed universal screening for AIDS and prescribes that if the "AIDS test" [there is no such thing as an AIDS test] is positive, that person "should be tattooed in the upper forearm, to protect common-needle users, and on the buttocks, to prevent victimization of other homosexuals" (Shelp & Sunderland 1987, 21).

Finally, political extremist Lyndon LaRouche's aptly named organization, The Prevent AIDS Now Initiative Committee (PANIC), successfully placed a proposition on the California ballot in 1986 that, if passed, could have barred infected people from certain jobs, mandated reporting infected persons to state health authorities, and possibly sanctioned the quarantining of PWAs, PWARCs, and PHIV+s (Shelp and Sunderland 1987, 22).

The flames of AIDS hysteria are being fanned by such uninformed reactions. AIDS hysteria is especially ugly because it helps generate even more ignorance and fear of the disease and increases the denial that prevents people from learning how the disease is spread; it contributes to homophobia, and alienates people from the PWA, PWARC, and PHIV + who need the support of their families, friends, and society. Next to AIDS, AIDS hysteria is possibly the most ugly disease from which a person can suffer.

Contamination, Alienation, and Discrimination

Although AIDS is not easy to "catch" (see chapter 1), the fear of AIDS contamination, whether rational or irrational, produces an enormous amount of alienation and discrimination.

The PWA, PWARC, or PHIV +, even in a relatively healthy relationship, suffers greatly due to others' fear of contamination. The AIDS Project staff at the Ackerman Institute in New York City noted that many of the couples they are working with avoid sex after an AIDS diagnosis in one of the partners. They have found that there is an inextricable connection between disease and contamination.

The FWA, especially the family of origin or family of choice that has assumed responsibility for the PWA's primary health care, must live with a daily fear of contamination. This can be a reasonable apprehension of accidental contact with the AIDS patient's body fluid in a cut or open sore or an irrational but real fear of contamination from household articles (for example, an unwashed glass).

Unfortunately, the fear of contagion (in many cases an irrational fear) is not reserved to the gay couple or the FWA. It has spread to the health care profession. It is not uncommon to hear of doctors who will not treat PWAs, nurses who will not care for them, housekeepers who will not clean their rooms, dietitians who will not bring the food tray into the room, and chaplains who visit from the hallway if they visit at all.

As the PWA watches his life begin to slip away, others' fear of catching the disease from him may make him feel that he will have to face the AIDS crisis alone.

This fear of being contaminated spawns a terrible response from society. The PWA, PWARC, PHIV +, and FWA often become victims of discrimination from a variety of sources and in a variety of ways, many of which are illegal if not immoral:

1. *Medical services.* The PWA, PWARC, PHIV+, and his family are particularly vulnerable within the medical system because an AIDS-related diagnosis will almost always demand a great deal of medical attention.

Doctors, dentists, and other licensed health care professionals in New York state are not required by law to accept a PWA, PWARC, or PHIV+ in their practice. However, professional codes of ethics require that practitioners not "abandon" the PWA, PWARC, or PHIV+ without first making alternative arrangements for "adequate care" by another practitioner. Although there may be sound medical reasons for a physician to do this, it is difficult to believe that discrimination is not one of the major factors at work when this happens. However, the law does require that ambulance services and hospital personnel provide care for the PWA, PWARC, and PHIV+. Nevertheless, the patient can experience discrimination in the hospital when (*a*) he is isolated far beyond the degree necessary to protect others from infection or to protect him from infection; (*b*) hospital personnel refuse to bathe the patient, enter his room with a meal tray, or clean his room; and, especially in the case of gay men, (*c*) hospital personnel restrict visitors who are not members of the family.

2. *Confidentiality.* Because of the stigma attached to AIDS and the discrimination that this stigma nurtures, the PWA, PWARC, or PHIV+ has a strong investment in protecting the confidentiality of his diagnosis and medical records. This can be a potentially dangerous area for discrimination. Disclosure of this kind of information can mean the loss of a job and a place to live, the denial of a loan or an insurance policy, the withholding of medical care and, if the person is an alien, even deportation. It is no surprise that many people affected with this disease are sensitive to any form of discrimination that might compromise their need for confidentiality. A few states already have a case-reporting system, which includes a mandatory contact-tracing policy by which PWAs would have to reveal all of their sexual contacts and be subject to selective quarantine. Subsequently, people who are at risk for the HIV virus often feel most secure in being tested at an anonymous site where the results will be identified by a code number, not a name.

3. *Personal matters.* The gay PWA, PWARC, or PHIV + may also feel discrimination in personal matters related to his financial or business assets and obligations. He should consider having a will for at least two reasons: first, the erratic nature of the disease can result in dementia and even death without much warning; and second, if the PWA, PWARC, or PHIV + dies without a will, the state does not recognize ties of affection (for example, to a lover). Whatever property is left will go to the next of kin, by birth or marriage. Without a will, the lover or the gay "family of choice," who may have assumed 100 percent of the financial and emotional obligations for the PWA's health care, can be left penniless and even homeless. This can be even more painful if the family of origin discriminates against the PWA's lover after his death.

4. *Insurance.* With the rapidly increasing number of AIDS cases and the escalating cost of medical care for AIDS patients, insurance companies are becoming increasingly reluctant to cover people whom they perceive to be at "high risk" for AIDS. The PWA, PWARC, or PHIV + may feel this form of discrimination in various ways. For instance, an insurance company may (a) refuse to insure him in the first place; (b) increase his payments or cancel his policy; (c) refuse to upgrade a policy thereby preventing an increase in benefits; or (d) pursue a policy of "redlining" all single men between the ages of twenty-five and forty-five. This is also an issue for the "worried well" because, if the insurance company perceives the applicant to be "at risk," it may require a blood test to determine if the applicant has been exposed to the HIV virus.

5. *Employment.* People with AIDS, ARC, who test HIV +, or those perceived to be "at risk" (for example, gay men) often encounter employment discrimination: dismissal; rejection of job applications; isolation at the workplace; being "loaned out" to a charitable organization (as a tax break and a way to keep other employees content); being forced to take an unpaid leave or a medical discharge. For those who seek employment, discrimination may take the form of a mandatory HIV test as a screening device.

The PWA, PWARC, or PHIV + might also be let go by an employer who claims to be upholding the law requiring him to provide a "safe working environment" for his or her employees. This rationale may be used to dismiss a person even though the Center for Disease Control has declared that there is no risk of contagion through normal working place contacts that occur among employees or between workers and clients or customers (*Living with AIDS* 1987, 1–30).

This long and depressing list of discrimination can be lengthened to include neighbors who will no longer talk to the PWA, PWARC, PHIV +, and his family; members of the clergy who represent religious traditions that offer little compassion if not condemnation; funeral homes that will not bury the body or charge more to do so; and a political system that has been accused of responding too slowly with too little.

The Double-Barrel Effect

Many PWAs, PWARCs, and HIV + s must face the double disclosure of telling their families of their HIV diagnosis *and* their sexual orientation. Either one of these issues can be difficult for the parents and siblings to deal with. Both of them can be devastating. Such a double-barreled disclosure can limit the FWA's ability to discuss the matter with their son and brother as well as interferes with their willingness to lend support. Time and time again, the hospitalized PWA would say "Now I not only have to tell my parents that I am gay, I also have to tell them that I am dying!"

The power of such a disclosure can result in a unique form of rejection. The discrimination that a gay PWA confronts can be doubled by the possibility that even his family may discriminate against him.

> A black family certainly isn't going to reject a daughter who is proud of being an Afro-American. An Hispanic family isn't going to abandon a son who is being treated badly at work because of his ethnic background. But gay people face probable rejection here [from the family], too. They usually end up being isolated on both fronts (Fortunato 1982, 35).

This is a horrible circumstance because the double barrel of this gun points in two directions: the family and the gay PWA,

PWARC, or PHIV +. Everyone has so much to lose. The gay PWA, PWARC, or PHIV + is threatened with the loss of his family and his life. The FWA must consider losing an image of their son as well as the son. The stress that this kind of revelation can produce in a family is hard to imagine.

Denial

AIDS is most often caused by behavior many people do not participate in or find reprehensible: IV drug use, multiple sex partners, and anal sex. Consequently, there is a tendency to deny the problem of AIDS because AIDS, by virtue of its sexual mode of transmission, is perceived to be repugnant to monogamous, heterosexual people. This attitude will change as AIDS continues to move into the heterosexual community; presently the prevalence of denial is keeping AIDS at a distance. This distance only complicates the problem because many people know too little about how the disease is spread and therefore have not taken it as seriously as it should be taken.

There is a positive form of denial when it comes to AIDS, and this is important for people in the therapeutic community to understand. "Healthy" denial, a denial that keeps some issues at a distance until the person is ready to deal with them, can help the PWA, PWARC, or PHIV + and his family deal with the plethora of psychosocial stressors at a more reasonable pace. If a person has to confront the disease and the psychosocial stressors that gather around it all at once, he may be unable to handle the pressure. Persons affected by AIDS need to deal with the issues one at a time and at a rate that will not throw them into dysfunction.

Finances

It would be futile to try to estimate the financial burdens that AIDS will lay upon the PWA, PWARC, PHIV +, his family, and society in general. With every new press release comes an escalated estimate of the cost per person that this disease will put on the national health care system. Practically no one will be able to hand the medical, pharmaceutical, clinical, therapeutic, home care, or hospital expenses that AIDS incurs. Almost everyone with a diagnosis of AIDS will need to depend on federal or state subsidized programs to assist him. No matter how much local, state, or federal assistance a person might receive, there will always be a list of needs that will not be covered or are required before they can be procured through the appropriate systems.

The PWA, PWARC, or PHIV+ will often see his life savings exhausted, only to learn that he is, with all his insurance benefits and government assistance, still a financial burden to families and friends.

Physical and Emotional Confusion

Having AIDS can be like a roller coaster ride. Physically speaking, a PWA or PWARC can be healthy one day, hospitalized the next, on his deathbed within the week, and discharged a few days later. Emotionally speaking, a PWA, PWARC, or FWA can be preparing for death on Friday and taking their son or lover home on Monday. These scenarios can be repeated time and time again. This cycle can cause an enormous amount of confusion for the PWA or FWA. It is difficult enough to face one's own death the first time, but, having to do that two or three times can leave the PWA emotionally exhausted. The same holds true for the FWA. It is not uncommon to hear a parent or a lover admit, in a moment of weakness, that they wish the PWA would "just go ahead and die" because they can no longer take the strain of watching the disease push him to the brink of death only to give a reprieve until another opportunistic disease brings the PWA to the brink of death for the second or third time. The FWA will often be torn between the joy that this could be a remission and the anger that they and the PWA will only have to suffer through this trauma another time, possibly in the very near future.

Psychological Problems

In addition to emotional stresses, there can also be psychological problems when, either directly or indirectly, AIDS affects the central nervous system. This process can lead to confusion, seizures, dementia, and depression. The counselor must have some basic knowledge of the effects of this disease on the PWA's personality. This is not always an easy task because these biological problems can also be symptoms of psychological depression.

The central nervous system of the PWA is particularly vulnerable for three reasons. First, the AIDS virus affects both the lymphatic and nervous systems. Therefore, there can be direct HIV infection of the brain. Second, as the PWA's immune system weakens, his or her brain is more vulnerable to being infected by opportunistic diseases of the central nervous system. Third, the medication that the PWA is taking may have adverse affects on his or her brain.

AIDS Dementia Complex (ADC) is the most common neurological diagnosis in AIDS patients.

> AIDS Dementia Complex is often marked by initially subtle cognitive or behavior dysfunction occurring over weeks to months. Patients initially report memory loss, difficulty in concentrating, social withdrawal, and lethargy. Those early signs may often be attributed to depression and may be ignored until they eventually progress to more dramatic deficits involving severe dementia and psychomotor retardation. Motor disturbances initially include loss of coordination, tremors and unsteady gait, and may lead to severe ataxia and paraplegia (Selwyn 1986, 39).

Pastoral counselors or caregivers will need to be especially sensitive to the confusion that can be caused by this frightening phenomenon as well as the dread of this diagnosis that haunts the PWA, PWARC, or PHIV + and his family.

Chapter 4

FAMILY SYSTEMS THEORY

The family system theory developed by Murray Bowen can be one of the most appropriate methodologies available to help the family with AIDS (FWA) to deal with the plethora of psychosocial stressors accompanying this illness. This theory posits a systemic approach that is a radical change from the traditional cause-and-effect way of thinking about dysfunction in families. Family systems theory believes that the human person is not merely an autonomous individual who controls his or her own destiny. Rather, the person is intimately connected to his or her family, those around him or her, and his or her multigenerational past. Therefore, an individual's emotional or physical illness is viewed as the product of a total family problem.

This approach of family systems theory offers a valuable alternative to the traditional one-on-one work occurring between a therapist and a patient when that patient is in a life-threatening situation like AIDS (Walker 1987a, 1). Professionals who usually see only one part of the family system begin to see the significant others in the client's life through the client's eyes. Ignorance of what actually takes place in the family may promote sympathy for what is going on in the family rather than assistance in helping the client change his or her relationship to the family and his or her role in the family. The family systems approach is also valuable for the therapist because, by soliciting the assistance of family members, it reduces some of the burn-out producing pressure of working with people suffering with a life-threatening disease.

Whether the family therapist is working with the family of origin, the family of choice, or a combination of the two, the important presumption is that a person with AIDS (PWA), with AIDS Related Complex (PWARC), or with Human Immunodeficiency Virus (PHIV+) needs the acceptance and support of his "family" to deal with a disease that has been so aptly labeled the "plague that lays waste at noon" (Fortunato 1985, 6). This chapter will introduce the elements of family systems theory that seem to be most applicable to working with persons with AIDS and their families.

This description of family systems theory ideally will encourage the reader to pursue this methodology because it dovetails so well with ministry. However, such a brief discussion can only be an introduction. If the reader is interested in family therapy, he or she must follow up that curiosity with an in-depth study of psychotherapy from the systematic point of view.

Differentiation of Self

Unconvinced that emotional illness was just the product of forces of socialization and specific only to humans, Murray Bowen did extensive reading in evolution, biology, and the natural sciences as part of a search for clues that could lead to a broader theoretical frame of reference (Bowen 1978, 353). From this study Bowen concluded that the emotional system governs the "dance of life" in all living things. The steps of this "dance" are found in the natural evolutionary past and are much older than the intellectual system. Therefore, feelings derive from the deeper emotional system. Bowen postulates that far more human activity is governed by the human's emotional system than people are willing to admit, and that there is far more similarity than dissimilarity between the way human forms and lower forms act.

Consequently, Bowen suggests that emotional illness is due to the adverse influence of the emotional system on the intellectual system and that severe forms of emotional illness are caused by a "flooding" of the intellectual system, thus resulting in emotional dysfunctioning. The subsequent "fusion" between the emotional and the intellectual can happen by degrees. The greater the fusion, the more the person's life is governed by the autonomic emotional forces within himself or herself, and the greater the fusion with the emotional systems of other people around the person. Bowen also believes that the greater the fusion, the more the person is susceptible to physical illness, emotional illness, and social illness, and the less the person is able to control his or her own life. However, it is possible for one to discriminate between the emotions and the intellect and slowly gain more conscious control of emotional functioning. The biofeedback phenomenon is an empirical example of conscious control over autonomic functioning (Bowen 1978, 304–5).

The core of Bowen theory has to do with the degree to which people are able to distinguish between their "feeling" system and their "thinking" system. Bowen says the emotional system is a carryover from the person's more primitive origins, while the intellectual system represents the human person at the pinnacle of his or her power (Paolino and McCrady 1978, 331). Thus the degree to which feelings and thoughts are fused or differentiated leads to the central concept of his theory: the "differentiation of the self."

> Differentiation means the capacity of a family member to define his or her own life's goals and values apart from surrounding togetherness pressures, to say "I" when others are demanding "you" and "we." It includes the capacity to maintain a (relatively) nonanxious presence in the midst of an anxious system, to take maximum responsibility for one's own destiny and emotional being. It can be measured somewhat by the breadth of one's repertoire of responses when confronted by a crisis (Friedman 1985, 27).

In order to understand fully the application of this concept, it is important to know that his theory deals with two kinds of variables, those relating to anxiety and those relating to the differentiation of the self. Bowen writes:

> There are several variables having to do with anxiety or emotional tension. Among these are intensity, duration, and different kinds of anxiety. There are far more variables that have to do with the

level of integration of the differentiation of self. This is the principle subject of this theory. All organisms are reasonably adaptable to acute anxiety. It is sustained or chronic anxiety that is most useful in determining the differentiation of self. If anxiety is sufficiently low, almost any organism can appear normal in the sense that it is symptom free. When anxiety increases and remains chronic for a certain period, the organism develops tension, either within itself or in the relationship system, and the tension results in symptoms or dysfunction or sickness. The tension may result in physiological symptoms or physical symptoms, in emotional dysfunction, in social illness characterized by impulsiveness or withdrawal, or by social misbehavior (Bowen 1978, 361–62)

The therapeutic method that grows out of this insight is based on two assumptions: (1) that reduction of anxiety in the emotional field will improve the functional level of differentiation of self and reduce symptoms; and (2) that improvement in the basic level of differentiation will increase the adaptability of the person to intense emotional fields. These perceptions are especially important to the PWA whose immune system may be more vulnerable to anxiety and stress (not to mention the myriad of psychosocial factors listed in chapters 2 and 3), and the FWA, especially if family members are at a lower level of differentiation.

Michael E. Kerr, coauthor with Bowen of *Family Evaluation*, points out that the "greater this fusion or lack of differentiation between the intellectual and emotional systems, the greater the influence of the togetherness life force on a person's functioning" (Gurman and Kniskern 1981, 238). This togetherness is manifest in a variety of ways. The best measure of the influence of this togetherness factor is the degree to which a person's thinking, feeling, and actions are dependent on or influenced by the emotionality of other people. This can take shape in two opposite but equally undifferentiated ways: overt emotional dependence (seeking approval, being dependent, pleasing others, feeling obliged, and conforming to what the other seems to want), or reactive withdrawal (seeking disapproval and rebelling against the perceived wishes of the other). These reactions are opposite sides of the same coin and, therefore, part of the same togetherness influence. This emotional reactivity of people to each other produces the emotional pressure people feel from each other to think and act in specified ways. When the intellectual and emotional systems are fused and there is a pronounced togetherness orientation in a person, we can expect to see more difficulty coping with or keeping an emotional balance; an impaired ability to be aware of and express feelings in an appropriate way; poor definition of boundaries between self and others, such as an obligatory sense of responsibility for the emotional well-being of another person, or the expectation that someone else is responsible for one's emotional well-being; unrealistic assessments of oneself and others; a dogmatic adherence to ideas and opinions in an authoritarian way; and a selfishness that may respect the boundaries of the self but fails to respect the boundaries of others (Gurman and Kniskern, 1981, 237–39).

Another clarification that is helpful when dealing with the complicated notion of differentiation is a delineation between what Paolino calls "intra-individual" differentiation (Paolino and McCrady 1978, 521) versus the "interpersonal" side of differentiation that deals with an individual's need to become autonomous yet still connected to his or her family of origin. If we look at differentiation at these two levels, perhaps the theory and application will be more clear.

Intra-Individual Differentiation of Self

The level of intra-individual differentiation is marked by the ability to separate feeling from thinking. A poorly differentiated person can hardly distinguish thoughts from feelings. The well-differentiated person is not one who only thinks and never feels but rather one who is able to balance thinking and feeling, capable of having strong emotions and spontaneity but equally capable of restraint so as not to act on emotional impulses (Nichols 1984, 350).

Kerr suggests looking at this phenomenon in terms of "basic" and "functional" differentiation. Basic differentiation reflects a person's average ability to keep intellectually and emotionally based functioning distinct and the power to retain choice about which system influences his or her activity in a given situation. After the level of basic differentiation is set, changes in it are uncommon except through systematic efforts to make them. Basic differentiation aligns with Bowen's idea about the "solid self." The solid self refers to that part of the individual that is non-negotiable under pressure from the relationship system. A solid self person would respond to emotionally charged situations by saying: "This is who I am and what I believe and this is the point beyond which I will not go." The emotional pressures of the group will not affect a well-differentiated solid self; consequently, a solid self will stand on his or her own two feet.

Functional differentiation relates to the degree of fusion between the intellectual and emotional systems that is influenced by the day-to-day shifts in the level of anxiety that a person experiences. Bowen uses the concept of "pseudoself" to describe this facet of individuation. A pseudoself can look like a solid self, but the clue that the person is not a solid self is the presence of a discrepancy between what a person says he or she does and what he or she actually does when under pressure from the relationship system. The pseudoself is negotiable, which is to say it can be changed under pressure. Such a person at a low functional level of differentiation is one whose life is floundering and who may be experiencing significant physical or emotional symptoms. For instance, if such a person gets married, joins a cult, or establishes a homosexual relationship, this person may, as a result of a relationship fusion with the other(s), begin to function better. This is a functional and not a basic change in differentiation because it depends on the relationship fusion to sustain it (Gurman and Kniskern 1981, 247–48).

Bowen developed the scale of differentiation to illustrate the principles for estimating the degree of fusion between the intellect and emotions. The term "scale" conveys the idea that people are different from each other and that this difference can be estimated from clinical information. Bowen does not intend this scale to be used as a psychological instrument for testing, but as an evaluation tool. This scale eliminates the concept of "normal" and has nothing to do with emotional illness or psychopathology. Nor does the scale have any direct correlation with intelligence or socioeconomic levels.

The chart and profiles following will summarize the detailed theory of differentiation.

low 0 – – – – 25 – – – – 50 – – – – 75 – – – – 100 high

In between "low" and "high" are an infinite number of mixes between emotional and intellectual functioning.

0 to 25 Range or Low Level of Differentiation. This person finds it impossible to distinguish feeling from fact. He or she is so totally relationship oriented that an enormous amount of energy goes into seeking love and approval. Consequently, there is no energy left for life-directed goals. A person with such a low level of differentiation of self might remain very dependent upon his or her parents or develop an equally dependent relationship with a significant other.

25 to 50 Range or Moderate Level of Differentiation. At this point of self-knowledge, a person discovers an ability to differentiate between the emotional and intellectual systems with most of the self expressed as a "pseudoself." However, there is enough flexibility to allow an interplay between emotionality and intellect. Therefore, when anxiety is low this person can function at a level that resembles good differentiation.

50 to 75 Range or Good Level of Differentiation. The hallmark of this person is that he or she is differentiated enough for the emotional and intellectual systems to function alongside each other without fusion. When anxiety increases, this person's intellectual system, unlike that of the two preceding groups, can hold its own. The intellect is no longer a "pretend" intellect that only gives the appearance of autonomy when anxiety is low. This person has a more "solid self" and therefore lives life more freely and has a more satisfying emotional life.

75 to 100 Range or High Level of Differentiation. This person is operationally clear about the difference between feeling and thinking. It is as routine for him or her to make a decision on the basis of well-integrated thinking as it is for a low-level person to make a decision based on feeling. On the level of intimacy, such a person is free to lose "self" in the intimacy of a close relationship without any fear of fusion or pursuing that relationship just because of needs. Bowen wants us to understand that this person is not a "rugged individualist," for he considers such a person to be the exaggerated pretend version of a person struggling against emotional fusion. Rather, the well-differentiated person is always aware of others and the relationship system around himself or herself (Bowen 1978, 370).

Once the self has been differentiated internally, only half of the process has been completed. Now attention has to be given to the person in the context of his or her family system.

Differentiation of Self from the Family of Origin

Probably one of the most central theoretical premises of family systems theory is the significance of the degree of a person's unresolved emotional attachments to his or her family of origin. This concept grew out of the realization that no matter how much people denied it or pretended to be separate from their family of origin, many people are still "stuck to" the members of their family and that "stuck togetherness" still continues to operate in the background of all their relationships. Bowen believes that the level of differentiation of a person is largely determined by the time one leaves home and attempts to live on one's own. Thereafter, the person tends to replicate the life-style from the family of origin in all future relationships (Bowen 1978, 371).

It becomes obvious how important it is for the individual to come to healthy terms with his or her differentiation from the family of origin. If a child is "selected" from among his or her siblings by virtue of birth position, gender, being born at a time of turmoil, being born with a defect or, in the case of this study, being a member of a sexual minority, the child may have an enormous project ahead of himself or herself in the process of differentiating from the family of origin. Interestingly enough, this process may include only one of many children, so that the oldest or youngest son, for example, may be caught in an intense emotional triangle in his family of origin while his other siblings are completely spared.

Family systems theory posits that in a tension field two people will predictably involve a third person to make a triangle. The lower the level of differentiation of self, the more intense the triangling process. And similarly, the higher the anxiety, the more intense the automatic triangling. When someone, usually the one in the most uncomfortable location in that triangle (such as the identified patient), tries to liberate himself or herself from that spot, the equilibrium (or homeostasis) of the triangle will be upset and those who prefer no change will rally to maintain the status quo and block any efforts to change the system. A person who is struggling to differentiate himself or herself in the family of origin must be well aware of this dynamic and, in particular, the process of detriangling.

Based on his own experience with his family of origin (Nichols 1984, 54), Bowen discovered that the most important primary triangle in a person's life, and the one that forms a pattern for all other relationships, is the triangle between a self and parents. If a person's emotional attachments with his or her parents remain unresolved, he or she will be stuck at a lower level of differentiation of self than if he or she is willing to come to grips with those issues that keep him or her stuck.

Bowen describes a classic technique for detriangling oneself from one's family of origin (or, for that matter, from any system). When one parent reports information secretly about the other, a son or daughter finds himself or herself in the middle. The person can detriangle himself or herself by sharing information with one parent given by the other parent. This strategy can be very effective in keeping one's parents from trying to get one to take sides. For example, Bowen's parents were accustomed to complaining to him about unresolved tension and conflict in their relationship. Recognizing the triangulation and the permission his participation gave them not to face their own problems, Bowen moved himself out of the third position with quips like: "Your wife told me a story about you; I wonder why she told me instead of you" (Nichols 1984, 54).

When any family member makes a move toward differentiating a self, the family emotional system communicates a three-stage verbal and nonverbal message: (1) "you are wrong"; (2) "return to your former self" (such as from gay to straight); (3) "if you do not revert, these are the consequences." The differentiating person responds (1) with an intra-individual response that can include almost any emotional or psychological symptom or even symptoms of physical illness; or (2) by merging into the family's togetherness within hours; or (3) by fighting back, which is still part of the family reaction-response system. These reaction responses can include tactics such as silence, withdrawal, running away, vowing never to return again, and fusing into another receptive ("substitute") family only to duplicate old patterns in the new emotional field. Of course, there is still one more option and that is to continue the differentiation process.

The differentiating person would recognize that an emotional system responds to emotional stimuli and, therefore, if one can control one's emotional response, one can interrupt the chain reaction of events in the family. In order to do this, the differentiating person must know the triangles, develop an ability to observe and predict the chain-reaction events in the family, and control his or her own response to the system while remaining in constant emotional contact with the family. These differentiating steps require long and careful deliberation that will allow the person to interact with the family of origin without reverting to anger, attack, or debate; for one of these responses would only relocate the differentiating self back into the middle of the family's emotional system.

However, even with an understanding of all these factors, the differentiating person must still face the dragon of "togetherness forces" in his or her family. Armed with calm arguments, righteousness, fervent pleading, accusation, solicitousness, and even threats, the family's togetherness forces will try to thwart the person's quest for differentiation. Obviously, this is a time when the therapist is most important; it will be his or her job to help the differentiating person fend off the assaults of the togetherness dragon. A young man who is suffering from AIDS, ARC, or who tests HIV + and wants to maintain his autonomy from his family of origin, while at the same time receiving their help, is a challenge to any family systems coach.

When the differentiating person can control his or her emotional reactions and begin to function more and more out of his or her intellectual system, the family will reach an emotional showdown. However, if the person can stand on his or her own in the thick of the fight, the family anxiety and togetherness forces will subside and a new level of closeness will begin. This closeness will include an appreciation for the differentiating person, but it may also include an attempt on the part of the family of origin to focus on another person who is at an earlier stage of differentiating. Thus, the process may be duplicated unless the next potential victim is ready for the fight, or unless the family of origin has attained a higher level differentiation (Bowen 1978, 218).

The Extended, Multigenerational Family Field

The notion of the "extended, multigenerational family field" is a primary concept for Bowen's theory. From this perspective "family" consists of the entire kinship network of at least three generations, both as it currently exists and as it has evolved through time.

Three classic components of Bowen's theory that affect this extended, multigenerational family field are the "nuclear family emotional system," the "family projection process," and the "multigenerational transmission process."

The nuclear family emotional system deals with the emotional forces in families that operate over the years in recurrent patterns. This is the system that is responsible for the "cutting-off" of a family member with a low level of differentiation and his or her subsequent fusion in another relationship. This new fusion tends to produce one of the following: (1) a reactive emotional distance between partners; (2) physical or emotional dysfunction in one of the spouses; (3) overt marital conflict; or (4) projection of the problem onto one or more of the children (Nichols 1984, 351).

The family projection process occurs when parental problems (such as their immaturity and lack of differentiation) are projected onto the children. The basic pattern often involves a mother whose emotional system is more focused on children than on her husband and a father who is sensitive to his wife's anxiety and supports her emotional involvement with the children. Although a mother might work hard to treat all her children the same, because of the varying degree of emotional fusion with each child she will have one child with whom the fusion is far more intense. The intensely fused child may be the one who has a positive attachment to the mother, the one who was considered "strange" or different from infancy, or the one whom the mother rejected from birth and vice versa. This child becomes the "scapegoat" or "identified patient" who is chosen to carry the symptoms for the family of origin (Bowen 1978, 204–5).

The multigenerational transmission process defines the principle of projection when the process is repeated over a number of generations. This multigenerational phenomenon will produce children with higher, equal, or lower basic levels of differentiation from the parents. An example of this process would be a family that "produces" a child with a level of differentiation lower than that of the parents, that child later marries a spouse with an equal level of differentiation. This marriage produces a child with an even lower level, who, in turn, marries another with an equal level. That marriage produces a child with a still lower level of emotional functioning and the transmission process continues. According to this tenet of the theory, the most severe emotional problems (such as schizophrenia) are the products of such a process that has been at work lowering the levels of differentiation over several generations (Bowen 1978, 477).

All people function within the context of an "extended family field." This term includes the family of origin or the original nuclear family (parents and siblings) plus the other relatives (grandparents, aunts, uncles, cousins, brothers-in-law, sisters-in-law, nieces, nephews, wives, children, sons-in-law, daughters-in-law, grandchildren). Unlike traditional psychoanalytic counseling, which implies that only one's parents are important (and their importance is often relegated to the past), family systems theory professes that the entire network of the family is important and that it is important to the present as well as the past. In addition, the concept of the extended family field suggests that parents, even when they are adults, are someone else's children, and that they are still part of their own sibling systems, even after marriage.

The scope of this "extended family field" might lead one to conclude that Bowen would need an auditorium to do therapy with everyone who needs to be part of the process. Although it is possible that the family systems therapist might deal with more than one person, it is not necessary to have every aunt, uncle, and cousin involved in the process. Bowen believed that change is initiated by individuals (or couples) who are capable of affecting the rest of the family.

When one adheres to the extended family field concept, patterns become an important part of the therapeutic process. Issues like sex, money, alcohol, separation, health, etc., have an uncanny way of appearing and reappearing (Friedman 1985, 31). Therefore, the goal for the therapist is to look beyond the present problem and see issues in terms of the family projection process and the multigenerational transmission process. Before a client can make any headway into his or her family problems, he or she must comprehend how families do business. The cure is to go backwards, to visit parents, grandparents, aunts, uncles, etc., and learn how to get along with them (Nichols 1984, 388). To aid in identifying these patterns, Bowen developed the genogram, which is a format for displaying in a graphic way a family tree showing information about family members and their relationships over at least three generations.

According to Bowen theory it is misleading to label families "normal" or "abnormal." Rather, he believes that families vary along a continuum, from emotional fusion to differentiation. Differentiation takes place when family members are independent yet connected, when anxiety is low, and when a person (for example, a gay person) is in good emotional contact with his own family of origin. The mature couple is one in which the partners do not reduce contact with their parents and siblings in order to reduce the anxiety and conflict that often comes from dealing with them. Since they do not lose contact with their families of origin, they do not deny the discord of their family of origin. By dealing with that discord in an appropriate way and with the appropriate people, they do not recapitulate it in other relationships. These well-adjusted people are able to separate thinking from feeling and can remain independent of and still connected to their nuclear and extended families (Nichols 1984, 354–55).

Differentiation is not a concept that is applied only to the individual, for the entire extended family can be more or less differentiated. And, similarly, the higher the level of differentiation in an entire extended family, the healthier the system. In the case of a family with a male homosexual member, it is logical to conclude that the better able the family is to accept the homosexual member's preference, the more likely it will be that (1) this member will not be cut off; (2) he will not be "scapegoated" or "triangled" into an unstable dyad somewhere else in the extended family of origin; and (3) there will be less stress-producing anxiety in the life of the PWA, PWARC, and PHIV +.

The Emotional Cut-off

According to systems theory, one of the most significant and relatively predictable "life patterns" is the "emotional cut-off," or as it is sometimes called, the "cut-off."

The emotional cut-off is Bowen's way of describing the emotional distance between family members (such as a homosexual man and his family of origin) achieved by internal mechanisms or by physical distance. "Out of sight, out of mind" does not work when it comes to self-knowledge and one's family of origin. Running away does not resolve the connections between a child and his parents. According to Bowen's theory, the more intense the cut-off between a person and his parents, the more likely he is to repeat the same pattern in his future relationships.

All people have an emotional attachment to their parents that is more intense than most permit themselves to believe. The issue is not the existence of the attachment but how intense and unresolved the attachment is. Bowen believes that the mother-child relationship is the most common location for unresolved issues for both male and female children. Some adult children exhibit this behavior by living within the parental emotional field. There are those who consciously deny the unresolved attachment while living near the parents and others who cut-off from parents and leave home never to return or communicate with them again. Then there are those who cut-off from their own parents and append themselves to the families of their spouse or partner in their search for an "idealized family of origin." Lastly and possibly most common are those who partially cut-off from their family of origin by living away while maintaining a token contact with parents. However, the bottom line remains the same. Denied emotional attachments to the past are repeated in future relationships (for example, with wife, children, or lovers). Bowen's theory also proposes that the more one denies attachment to the past, the less choice one has in determining the pattern of his relationships. Bowen proposes that a relationship breakdown (such as threats to divorce, or emotional problems in the child of a heterosexual couple or threats of separation in a homosexual couple) is evidence of an unresolved emotional attachment to the family of origin (Bowen 1978, 433).

Staying home and being emotionally dependent on the family of origin or running away from the family are opposite sides of the same coin. Those who choose either "solution" equally need emotional closeness yet are equally allergic to it. The one who remains on the scene handles the attachment by intrapsychic mechanisms. He or she would be more apt to develop internalized symptoms under stress, such as physical illness or depression; social dysfunction, such as drinking and episodic irresponsibility in relation to others (Bowen 1978, 382). The higher the anxiety in the environment, the more one isolates himself or herself from others emotionally, while still appearing to carry on normal relationships in the group.

The "independent" person who runs away geographically (such as the "mobile" homosexual male) is more inclined to impulsive behavior (Bowen 1978, 536). Bowen suggests that in the case of an intense geographic cut-off, the person is more likely to duplicate that pattern with the first available person. As an example of this in the heterosexual community, Bowen cites an impulsive marriage followed by multiple marriages followed by temporary living-together relationships (Bowen 1978, 382). In the homosexual male community, it is fair to suspect there is a parallel phenomenon in which the intensely cut-off person moves from one sexual partner to another in his search for a loving relationship. Unfortunately such behavior contributes to the spread of venereal diseases such as AIDS (Bowen 1978, 382).

To further complicate the picture, the mobile, cut-off, homosexual male may be exposed to a kind of "undifferentiated society ego mass." Before industrialization, people were able to use physical distance to relieve the tension of emotional fusion. However, society has developed into a human mass where the individual, in this case the cut-off homosexual male, may become as alienated from his fellow humans as he was in his undifferentiated family ego mass. On a societal level, Bowen believes that promiscuous sexuality may be a panicky response to overcome the alienation of too much fusion to others (Bowen 1978, 440). This phenomenon would be more prevalent among homosexual men who opt to live in large urban areas where a countercultural sexual life-style is more available and more acceptable. The consequence of this is a pattern that may contribute to multiple sex partners, a behavior that can promote AIDS.

A different but related facet of the cut-off process is the role that secrets (underground or irresponsible communications) can play. Unlike the medical and individual psychotherapeutic models where confidentiality is an essential quality, family systems theory believes that there are situations in which keeping the confidence of one family member can be detrimental to the total family. This is based on the belief that the higher the level of anxiety and symptoms in a family, the more that family members are emotionally isolated from each other. Of course this can exacerbate the cut-off process that may already be in play with the family of a homosexual person. The greater the isolation, the lower the level of responsible communication between family members, and the higher the level of irresponsible underground gossip about each other in the family and the confiding of secrets to those outside the family. When a therapist pledges confidence, he or she gets pulled into the emotional network of the family. This can turn up the heat under the relationship problem, thereby complicating and extending the therapy and wasting time with the keeping of "secrets" under the pretense of confidentiality. The goals of a family therapist are to (1) reduce the level of anxiety; (2) improve the level of responsible open communications within the family; (3) reduce the irresponsible, underground communications of secrets (for example, gossip) to others; and (4) to know the difference between irresponsible, underground secrets and valid, responsible, private communications. Put more simply, the goal of a family therapist is to bridge cut-offs (Bowen 1978, 291).

Although Edwin H. Friedman does not mention closeted homosexuality among his list of subjects of secrets, he does point out that it really is not the content of the secret that is most significant but the "ramification of its existence for the emotional process of the entire family" (Friedman 1985, 52). Secrets, he claims, divide families into those who know and those who do not know. Those who are "in" on the secret will be far better at communicating with one another than with those in the outside group, not just about the secret, but about any issue. Secrets cause unnecessary estrangements as well as false companionship and distort perceptions because family members become confused or misled by information they receive. They think they are seeing the whole picture, yet they are seeing only a part. The most powerful effect of secrets on a family's emotional system is that they exacerbate other pathological processes unrelated to the content of the particular secret. Secrets generally function to keep anxiety at high energy levels, so, when secrets are revealed, the anxiety level of the family generally decreases (Friedman 1985, 52–53).

For the family therapist, aiding a person to recognize the existence of a relationship or the importance of reestablishing a relationship with the two or three generations of his family can be an important symptom-reducing influence (Gurman and Kniskern 1981, 250). Such an intervention can also be a significant influence in changing behavior. If the previously cut-off person is reconnected to his family of origin in a healthy way and begins to get some of his emotional needs met there, it follows that he may become less cut-off, less anxious, and less apt to move from relationship to relationship. If, because of the sexual revolution, moving from one relationship to another is more apt to include sex, and if having multiple sex partners is one of the major factors for the spread of AIDS, and if multiple reinfection is one of the significant factors that turns an HIV+ person into a PWARC or PWA, *then* dealing with emotional cut-off is a major therapeutic goal in the age of AIDS.

Person-to-Person Relationships

The opposite of a cut-off is a person-to-person relationship. "In broad terms, a person-to-person relationship is one in which two people can relate subjectively to each other and about each other, without talking about others (triangling), and without talking about objective 'things' " (Bowen 1978, 549). On a more practical level, a person-to-person relationship is one established between two fairly well differentiated people who can communicate directly, with respect for each other, and without the complications found between people who are less mature (Bowen 1978, 540). Bowen strongly suggests that a person-to-person relationship with each member of one's extended family will help that person individuate more than any other technique that could be prescribed. When an individual has a person-to-person relationship with as many members of his or her family as possible he or she can spread out his or her emotional energy instead of concentrating all emotional energy in one or two family relationships. Furthermore, since people learn how to relate to their families during childhood, people often relate to them as children. Because so many people leave their families before they have developed adult personalities, it is obvious that these same people can continue to react childishly to parents, brothers, sisters, etc. Returning to the family as an adult, in mature person-to-person relationships, enables the person to understand and modify his or her old relational patterns and begin to function as a differentiated adult (Nichols 1984, 364–65).

Another obstacle to establishing one-to-one relationships with parents is the myth of "parental we-ness." According to Bowen, one of the major misconceptions about child rearing is the idea that parents should present a united front in their child raising so that the child will not be able to play one against the other. Bowen feels that this is an unhealthy myth in three ways: (1) It prevents the child from knowing men inasmuch as he or she does not have a relationship with an individual man, that is, the father. Of course, the same is true for having a relationship with a woman. (2) From the standpoint of triangles, parental we-ness locks a child into a two-to-one triangle that provides no flexibility unless the child can manage to force a rift in the other side of the triangle. (3) Parental we-ness is an invitation for poorly differentiated parents to fuse into a common self, or a "parental-we." So, in the interest of differentiation for the person in question, for his or her parents, and for the family itself, parental we-ness is of little or no service. The concept needs to be demythologized (Bowen 1978, 497).

Life Patterns vs. Open Relationships

According to Bowen's theory, a person is "programmed" into an emotional configuration very early in life and he or she is only able to shift up or down the scale of differentiation a few "degrees" from where his or her parents ranked. Therefore, if a person's parents were "stuck" (for example, with an unresolved emotional attachment) in a triangled relationship with their own parents, he or she will be equally stuck in a triangled relationship with them. The consequence of all this triangulation will be systems with a higher lever of overall anxiety. There is a way out of such a system, but it entails an "open" relationship system (the opposite of an emotional cut-off). "An open relationship system . . . is one of which family members have a reasonable degree of emotional contact with each other" (Bowen 1978, 537). This is not an easy process, Bowen notes, because openness by itself does not increase the level of differentiation in a family. Rather, openness reduces anxiety and a continued low level of anxiety permits a motivated family to begin slow steps toward better differentiation (Bowen 1978, 537).

Seeking a Substitute Family vs.
Controlling One's Own Reactivity

A variation of the running away scenario is the tendency to find a "good" family to substitute for a "bad" family of origin. How often does a homosexual male move away from home in order to find acceptance, only to end up with another man who may have come from an equally unaccepting family of origin? This not to say that the only reason homosexual men move away from home is to cut off and find a substitute family. Nonetheless, it would be equally naive to think that this search for acceptance is not an option for the person who may have felt like a second-class family member or even an outcast because of his "countercultural" sexual orientation. Unfortunately, in most cases, Bowen believes that the substitute family is of little or no help because the relationships with that new idealized family will eventually duplicate the person's relationship with his or her family of origin. For example, when the stress or anxiety of life increases, the person will cut-off from that social relationship (for example, the new, "improved" family substitute) and seek another. If this scenario is repeated often enough, it can result in isolation.

Rather than spending his or her life looking for the "perfect" family to substitute for the one he or she got stuck with, Bowen suggests that each person become a better observer and learn how to control his or her emotional reactivity. Even if no one becomes completely objective or gets to the point where he or she never reacts emotionally to family situations, it is still of value to learn more about the family through better observations. In this way the emotional reactivity is automatically reduced. Getting "outside" the family's emotional system is an excellent way to stop blaming other family members and get beyond the anger— two emotions that do not profit the differentiation process. These skills are also useful in all kinds of emotional snarls. This is not to say that every day will be an opportunity to practice such techniques; most of the time a person can live his or her life reacting with natural emotional responses. However, at time of great stress, these skills are essential to help a person back out of a situation, slow down one's own emotional reactivity, and make observations that will help one to control one's self in a stressful situation.

Chapter 5

APPLICATIONS OF
FAMILY SYSTEMS
THEORY

Family systems theory as developed by Murray Bowen can be very useful to the therapist in working with persons and families with AIDS. In this chapter we will consider some of the most direct applications in relationship to the extended family field, the differentiation of self, and the cut-off.

The Extended Family Field

Bowen has provided the therapeutic world with an invaluable service by broadening the base of therapy beyond the nuclear family to the extended family, past and present. The goals for the extended family are relatively clear; for once the option is conceded that people are embedded in a larger social context, it seems obvious what needs to be done: open the system (Nichols 1984, 363–64).

Ross Speck widens the circle to include the social "network" that is the "family" of neighbors and friends (Nichols 1984, 64). He believes that these people are also important because they constitute the social context and also provide what is available for the support and nurturance of people with problems. To include these neighbors and friends in the therapeutic circle is particularly important to the homosexual man who may have a partner or lover (Nichols 194, 363).

The value of widening the extended family field is based on the belief that people can help one another, and normally they do. Thus, broadening the extended family field is an important insight for the family system therapist in dealing with most issues, especially AIDS. No family systems therapist would ever think of excluding a spouse or in-laws from the big picture, so the male partner and intimate circle of homosexual friends of the person with AIDS (PWA), the person with AIDS Related Complex (PWARC), or the person with Human Immunodeficiency Virus (PHIV +) must also be included in the therapeutic process. However, the position and function of a "lover" or "gay family" do not often find their way into traditional family systems theory. Nevertheless, the ever-growing crisis of AIDS in the male homosexual community may lead therapists to include these critically important relationships.

Russel Haber proposes to open the extended family field to include other systems that impact on the family such as schools, the workplace, places of worship, agencies, previous therapists, medical professionals, cultural groups, and the like (Haber 1987, 269).

Haber claims that friends can act as consultants, bringing new information to the family. Considering the secrecy that surrounds homosexuality, parents are frequently ignorant of or intrigued by what happens in other families. Listening to a nonfamily member can help the family with AIDS (FWA) gain a perspective on how life works in other family systems. A son who is working to differentiate himself from his family of origin by cutting them off may be able to bring a gay friend into therapy. His friend's family can be a role model if they are better differentiated and therefore more accepting of their son's sexual orientation. This kind of support may help keep his stress down, his health up, and his immune systems more intact. The involvement of homosexual friends or lovers in the family therapy sessions can also challenge the notion that the family can provide all the resources needed for the PWA, PWARC, or PHIV + . Considering the psychosocial scope of AIDS and the needs that a PWA, PWARC, or

PHIV+ will have, enlarging the system in a way that allows other people to help can be essential.

The PWA, PWARC, or PHIV+'s friends or lover can be a source of positive peer pressure. When dealing with a disease that is so unpredictable and provides an emotional roller coaster ride for its victims, peer support can be invaluable.

And lastly, since the PWA, PWARC, or PHIV+'s relational patterns with his family are often replicated with his peers, dealing with issues like intimacy or distance in his peer relationships may indirectly change his relationships with his family of origin. If those changes are positive, and if improved relationships decrease stress, and if reduced stress is a benefit to the immune system, then a person whose immune system is compromised by AIDS can only benefit by extending the extended family field.

Gillian Walker, co-director of the Ackerman Institute AIDS Project, echoes many of Haber's insights in her work with FWA. She claims that professionals who see only one part of the family system begin to see the significant others in the patient's life through the client's eyes. If therapists are unaware of the interpersonal dance, they may find themselves sympathizing with the compelling series of complaints but not helping the PWA to change the interpersonal context. Therefore, the AIDS team at Ackerman Institute is highly sensitized to working with PWA, PWARC, or PHIV+, and their lovers. However, Walker cautions that there is a certain resistance to family therapy as a treatment modality, especially in the homosexual community. In the beginning, the homosexual PWA, PWARC, or PHIV+ may not be willing to involve his family of origin. His internalized homophobia may be exacerbated by his fear of contaminating others and the common belief that AIDS is a punishment from God for one's sexual orientation and life-style. Walker cautions the therapist that these feelings and the accompanying depression may necessitate working with the PWA or PWARC until he feels confident enough to invite others whom he fears may echo his own negative feelings.

Statistics on family acceptance of the gay man's disclosure of this sexual orientation indicate that approximately 50 percent of all families react with some negativity to the admission of homosexuality in a family member. Therefore, "coming out" can be frightening and dangerous, especially if the client's life is complicated by a diagnosis of AIDS, ARC, or HIV + . Therefore, the client and therapist may first need to work on establishing or maintaining good relationships with the homosexual PWA's "family of choice" (for example, his gay friendship network). If and when this is accomplished, the therapist may be more successful in connecting the PWA to his family of origin, knowing that he (1) has had a good experience with his "family of choice" (2) has received their acceptance and support; and (3) feels strong enough to take the risk of reconnecting with his family of origin.

In her work with PWA, PWARC, and PHIV + , Walker has noticed some resistance to couple therapy. This may be attributable to the PWA's fear that beneath his lover's "apparent" acceptance and compassion he may discover blame ("Did you infect me?") or anger ("Why did you have to get infected and ruin everything?"), the anger he secretly believes he deserves as punishment. Or even worse, the PWA, PWARC, or PHIV + may discover that his lover, in order to protect himself, may want to leave. On the other side, the lover may not want to enter therapy because he wants to protect his PWA, PWARC, or PHIV + partner from his ambivalent feelings about staying or leaving (Walker 1987a and 1987b).

Differentiation and Stress

One can argue that the PWA, PWARC, or PHIV + , because of the legion of stressful factors that affect him (see chapters 2 and 3), may be more acutely susceptible to stress than any other person with a life-threatening disease. Such stress seriously interferes with his immune system and therefore makes him more vulnerable to the opportunistic diseases that threaten his life. Therefore, the PWA may particularly need the kind of intervention that can aid him in reducing his level of stress, that is to say, family systems theory.

The person with a higher level of differentiation will be better able to deal with the emotionally volatile psychosocial issues that surround him. And, by the same token, the better differentiated the PWA, PWARC, or PHIV + is from his family of origin, the better his chances of staying in touch with the most suitable support group—his family.

Andrea Maloney-Schara proposes:

> If the development of AIDS is similar to the process in other families with life-threatening illness, then a generalized hypothesis can be constructed. The underlying assumption would be that the family as a unit forms automatic patterns of relationship which directly affect health. The hypothesis would be that an individual can increase his physiological and emotional functioning by lowering his overall level of arousal in order to change his functioning position in his family. The goal would be to increase the quality and length of a person's life by knowledge within the individual of the strengths and possibilities inherent in his biological and emotional relationship systems (Maloney-Schara 1987, 1).

Maloney-Schara states that this approach has been useful for a small sample of PWAs in the following ways: (1) it gives an individual factual evidence that he can influence his own physiology; (2) it can create a window of time to build in different behavioral responses to many seemingly threatening situations (such as the risk in trying to alter one's emotional position with one's family); and (3) the process of biofeedback can allow an individual the opportunity to examine his own beliefs while in a calm state. She believes that this increased ability of a PWA to reflect on the way in which he automatically operates can promote greater physiological flexibility and mental openness. This approach is rooted in the belief that the behavior of the organism is directed by a guidance system that is emotional, and that, over time, humans have learned more about the automatic nature of their responses. There is evidence to suggest that such awareness can lead to behavioral changes that promote health. The assumption is that the physiology of the individual, in this case of the PWA, PWARC, or PHIV+, is closely associated with the functioning of the emotional system.

A growing body of research in psychoneuroimmunology correlates emotional states and behavior responses with indicators of immune system function. Further research may reveal a range of flexibility in immune system functioning similar to what is currently seen with other physiological indicators.

The application is obvious: In the case of AIDS, ARC, or HIV positivity, it is possible to affect, within limits, the functioning of the immune system through biofeedback. Put more simply, improvement in one's ability to be oneself (for example, attaining a higher level of differentiation) or improvement in one's ability to adapt to others (for example, an improvement in one's differentiation from one's family of origin), could alter the immune system and make it more capable of fending off opportunistic diseases.

Harold Noer, a molecular biologist, points out that after exposure to the virus and confirmation of the presence of antibodies, there is an average latency of four to five years before the symptoms of ARC or AIDS appear. Exactly why someone progresses from a latent phase to an active phase is yet unknown. One explanation for this conversion is that some individuals in the latent phase have little or no free virus in their blood. Each time they develop a minor infectious disease, such as the flu, the virus is released into the bloodstream for a brief period of time. Then the amount of virus in the bloodstream returns to zero or to a low baseline. This process continues repeatedly until a point when the amount of the virus does not decrease after a release. This represents the critical shift from latent to active phase and the appearance of symptoms associated with ARC or AIDS. Therefore, Noer believes that the number of challenges that the immune system must contend with after exposure to the AIDS virus can be seen as part of the process hastening the development of clinical AIDS (Noer 1988, 5).

How then can a PHIV + minimize the effects of such challenges to the immune system and retard the change from latent to active phase of the process? Noer proposes that, although there may be several methods to accomplish this, the one that is most appropriate to family systems theory revolves around how a PHIV + can influence his own cellular system or immune system. Although classical physiology says that such an "influence" is not possible, recent research has shown that severe stress (for example, the kind of stress that can be caused by one or many of the psychosocial factors that surrounds AIDS) causes a decrease in the level of lymphocytes, the targets for the AIDS virus, and a decrease in the responsiveness of the lymphocytes to infectious bodies. Consequently, understanding how the body or the mind regulates the lymphocytes' responsiveness would be a major accomplishment in controlling the AIDS virus.

This research supports the assumption that stress reduction, accomplished by improving the level of differentiation of the self, and the differentiation of the self from the family of origin, can be positive therapeutic goals in dealing with PWA, PWARC, and PHIV +.

Maloney-Schara takes these ideas two steps further by proposing an application of these ideas to the individual in relation to his family and in relation to society. On the assumption that the individual has been "tuned" to react automatically in the early relationship system to which he is attached, she proposes that the development of symptoms reflects the anxious focus of the caretakers (in most cases, the family of origin). Therefore, the emotional and psychosocial stressors on the individual, discussed in chapters 2 and 3, and their affects on the immune system would be only one factor. The family of origin could be another contributing stress factor in the conversion from HIV positivity to ARC or AIDS. Maloney-Schara proposes that being the object of the negative focus in the family can affect both the functioning of the immune system and perhaps the activation of genetic predispositions. She says there is evidence that the focused-on person within the family is more vulnerable to development of emotional, physical, or social symptoms.

Maloney-Schara proposes that since society reflects the process that is within the family, then society can be a third factor in producing the kind of stress that psychoimmunology suggests can push the HIV + into ARC or AIDS.

When under higher levels of arousal (such as hysteria) the caretaker, whether it be the family or society, may act with less flexibility and even overreact to a situation. What better person or group of persons is there to receive this negative overreaction than homosexuals who have been perceived negatively by most cultures?

Therefore, stress for the PHIV + can come from self, family, or society. This evaluation should make family systems therapists even more sensitive to the plight of the PWA, PWARC, and PHIV +.

Differentiation and
Open Relationships

On the assumption that a crisis can be an opportunity to grow, it is advisable to work with a PWA, PWARC, or PHIV+ on raising his level of differentiation—even if it may not produce a significant improvement in his immune system and even if reconnecting with the family of origin is not possible or advisable. In fact, reconnecting at the wrong time, or with a family in which there are few prospects of positive results, will only add to the stress of the PWA, PWARC, or PHIV+, and thereby increase his stress and decrease the ability to deal with his family, and negatively affect his immune system.

The principles of differentiation of self along with an awareness of patterns in family history can be very useful when working with the PWA, PWARC, and PHIV+. They help visualize the "multigenerational transmission process," to surface issues, and aid the client in visualizing and verbalizing the concerns that he may bring into therapy or has come to face through therapy. Many of the psychosocial factors of this disease are major stresses, so there is never a lack of emotionally laden issues that need to be faced in an intellectual way in order to give the client more power over his life and a better chance at raising his level of differentiation.

Being a member of a sexual minority will be a significant factor since the position one holds in the family structure can influence one's functioning, relational patterns, and the type of relationships one will form in the next generation.

Since PWA, PWARC, and PHIV+ may be more vulnerable to stress than other people facing a life-threatening disease, the "flow of anxiety" that happens in every family is important to observe and chart. Whether the stress be "vertical," from one generation to the next, or "horizontal," across the family from current strain on the family as it moves through the life cycle, it can be beneficial for the PWA to see this process as he struggles to liberate himself from its adverse affects. "Coincidences" can be interpreted in a new way that will give the client the encouragement to do the hard work of differentiation. And, since the man who is a member of a sexual minority may be more apt to serve a dysfunctional purpose in his family of origin, helping him see fusion, enmeshment, conflict, cut-off, triangulation, and closeness could be beneficial for him.

Techniques from Bowen's theory for developing more open relationships would be appropriate for accomplishing such differentiation. And developing more open relationships is certainly one of the possibilities for a PWA, PWARC, or PHIV+, even if his family is not capable of bridging the emotional cut-off. Although Bowen does not see this process as a significant way of raising the level of differentiation, he admits that it can reduce anxiety in a family which might eventually begin to take slow steps toward differentiation. Therefore, one might be able to help a client ascend the scale of differentiation by enabling him to recognize how he is "stuck," for example, in a triangled relationship with his parents (who are similarly stuck in a triangled relationship with their parents), and by assisting the person to see how that enmeshment, or "stuck-togetherness," has programmed him to duplicate the same behavior of his parents and grandparents.

The first therapeutic goal for the PWA, PWARC, or PHIV+ would be to help him develop a more open relationship with his family of origin in which he and his family might share a reasonable degree of emotional contact.

A second issue that can be very appropriate to the homosexual community is the phenomenon of "substitute families." If it is fair to assume that many homosexual men feel unacceptable to their families of origin and therefore tend to cut-off, often with distance, then the therapist should be sensitive to the client who, in an attempt to establish some sense of family, connects with other men in the same situation. If a person is the victim of a cut-off pattern and is constantly seeking the approval and acceptance of a "good" family, this phenomenon may have something to do with the frequency of sex partners. A person who is searching for a new, improved family will duplicate the same behavior and encounter the same problems in each new relationship that he had in his family of origin. Therefore, each new relationship will fail with time, and he will move on to another. Since some of the obstacles to ending a relationship often do not exist in the homosexual community (such as children, shared property, legal concerns such as divorce, fear of family rejection, social stigma of divorce, etc.), the cut-off and substitute family process may be duplicated more rapidly. Consequently, these issues may be of greater concern for the PWA, PWARC, or PHIV + than for the general population.

A third, and one of the more frequent and powerful applications of family systems theory to the PWA, PWARC, and PHIV +, is the issue of "triangling" and the therapeutic intervention of "de-triangling."

Bowen theory proposes that the lower the level of differentiation of self, the more intense the triangling process and, similarly, the higher the anxiety, the more intense the automatic triangling. If the homosexual male or the homosexual male with AIDS, ARC, or who tests HIV + is in a particularly vulnerable position within the family, then the therapist would be wise to keep a sharp eye out for triangling.

If these assumptions are applicable and the PWA, PWARC, or PHIV + finds himself in the traditional "scapegoat" or "identified patient" position, then certain therapeutic techniques may be relevant. These would include: (1) helping the person to develop as many person-to-person relationships as possible within his family of origin (and, if necessary, outside his family of origin); (2) aiding him in developing a more open relationship system; (3) working with him on creating better observation skills; and (4) assisting him in developing his ability to control his own emotional reactivity. With such skills the triangled person will be better able to see the triangles in which he grew up and be better differentiated in relationship to them.

The Emotional Cut-off

Homosexual men seem to be susceptible to using the cut-off as a part of their development. The literature recounting the stories of homosexual men with AIDS, ARC, or who test HIV + is replete with incidents that illustrate the classic cut-offs. It is very common to read lines as: "Although he had been estranged from his mother and father for more than ten years . . ." (Bradley 1988, 46) and, "After several years, the hiding and the clandestine meetings began to take too much of a toll. The two lovers decided it was time to leave" (Bradley 1988, 37).

Some of the factors that may contribute to the tendency to cut off, especially by physical distance, might be (1) the general lack of societal acceptance of homosexuality and homosexual coupling; (2) the homosexual person fears that his sexual preference will engender feelings of failure in his parents; (3) some sexual activity of homosexual men may be considered unacceptable, illegal, or sinful (for example, anal intercourse); (4) men are often the targets of "homophobia," "homo-negativism," and "homo-confusion," which adds to feelings of alienation; (5) few religious bodies condone formal coupling for homosexual people; (6) the crisis of AIDS is saturated with issues of fear, and fear can add to the emotional temperature that can result in a cut-off. (Even in "accepting families," that is, those where some people know but the secret is kept from most of the family, there is often a limit to the acceptability of a homosexual relationship); (8) for those who choose to break the secret, "coming out" can be a painful process filled with the potential for rejection and loss; (9) homosexual people may feel attracted to other geographic locations because of their need for anonymity, their search for support from a broader-based gay community, the greater possibility of meeting people in a locality with a larger percentage of homosexual people, the improved chances for employment, etc.; (10) homosexual people, without the financial and relational restrictions of their heterosexual peers, often have more mobility.

If the process of leaving home for the homosexual man is or was colored by any of these issues, the family systems therapist will need to be alert to the issues that surround what could well be a developmental stage that has gone awry. A brief article found in *Family Therapy Today* offers some valuable suggestions about this process, especially if it is resolved by a cut-off. Sebastian Kraemer of the Child Guidance Training Centre in Whittington Hospital, London, suggests that the adolescent's leave taking is the "weakest link in the chain of family life and the one therefore to be broken if there is stress. Sometimes the difficulty is that the parents themselves have not emotionally left home" (*The Loss of Leaving Home*, 1986, 5). Therefore, in a situation such as a FWA, it may be advisable for the family systems therapist to take a close look at the circumstances surrounding the client's leaving home and the cutting-off process. Kraemer suggests asking questions such as: How old were you when you left home? How far from home did you go? What did your family know about where you were going? Had they seen where you would be living? Why did you leave at that particular time? Did you cook your own meals and do your own laundry? Were you the first sibling to leave home? What obligations persisted after you left? How often did you feel you should visit your family? (*The Loss of Leaving Home*, 1986, 5).

Gillian Walker, co-director of the Ackerman Institute's AIDS Project, has had an opportunity to apply family therapy to her work with PWAs. She confirms the need for sensitivity to the issue of cut-offs when she writes:

> In the gay community, gay couples are beginning to turn to therapists to help them handle their relationships when one or both are HIV-positive or have AIDS or ARC. Many are confused about how or if to tell their parents and families of origin about their diagnosis and about their homosexuality (Walker 1987a, 2).

Initial clinical impressions gathered from the beginning work with PWA, PWARC, and PHIV + show them to be people who are the products of fairly intense parent or child symbiosis and who have managed this intensity through fairly significant degrees of emotional cut-off. People who are most vulnerable are those who live with high levels of chronic anxiety that is managed mainly through relationships, in many instances homosexual relationships as well as with drugs and alcohol (Murphy 1988, 3).

Mary Ann Lancaster has proposed that families of origin of gay individuals manage their relationships in a number of ways, cut-offs being one of the most prevalent.

> In a study of 42 [male homosexual] patients at Memorial Sloan-Kettering Hospital, ⅓ lived alone and indicated the absence of a support network that would help them. Of the first 42 AIDS cases, 62% had either minimal or no contact with their families of origin. Often there are different patterns of communication among family members. Usually communication is most open with siblings and

least open with fathers. These patterns of communication contribute to confusion, ambivalence, and further isolation at a time of great emotional need. In general, families of origin of gay individuals manage family relationships in a number of ways including rejection, continued involvement without knowledge of the individual's homosexuality, ritualistic suppressed knowledge of lifestyle, and acceptance (Lancaster 1987, 20).

Andrea Maloney-Schara reminds us that, to some extent, the emotional cut-off is probably part of the way every family does business. In each family there are clear emotional patterns that are used to regulate the behavior of the various members. This regulation can be accomplished in two basic ways: (1) the person can be isolated or (2) negative attention (such as criticism) can be focused on the behavior that is unacceptable to the group while positive attention (such as praise) can be focused on behavior that is acceptable to the group. The purpose of this "regulation" is to produce conformity with the family. However, it tends to spin off a certain number of members who will be emotionally or geographically distant from the family, that is to say, cut-off. These emotional patterns are passed on from generation to generation and reflect a kind of ingrained blueprint that suggests what to look for in the behavior or appearance of the other person.

In the process of differentiation, the individuating person possesses an automatic emotional pattern that regulates his ability to hide his "self" from the other members of the family and blend in with the group. However, if a person is unable to find ways of differentiating himself from the family of origin, he may have difficulty in knowing who his "self" is. Thus the person has an increasing inability to distinguish himself from the family and greater difficulty in distinguishing his "self" from his "nonself." In keeping with classical family systems theory, Maloney-Schara proposes that one's inability to be a self in the family provokes an emotional or physical cut-off leaving the person more at risk. Put more simply, the more negative the family focuses upon an individual, the stronger the emotional cut-off will be; the stronger the emotional cut-off, the more removed from relationships one will be with significant others; the more removed from relationships with significant others, the more vulnerable the person becomes to the entire range of symptoms.

In the case of a family with a homosexual son, the more the son's sexual orientation is perceived as a stigma, the more the above equations will take effect. This also is an important understanding of the differentiation of the family of origin. The consequences are rather obvious: the more the family's negativity toward homosexuality, the less capable the homosexual PWA, PWARC, or PHIV+ is to promote his health or have his good health promoted by his family of origin; or, from the positive point of view, the more motivated the homosexual PWA, PWARC, or PHIV+ is to overcome the automatic way in which he and his family respond and react to each other by cutting-off, the greater chance he would have of improving his health. If a male homosexual with AIDS, ARC, or HIV+ can alter his functional position within his family of origin in a way that he can resolve his cut-off, he may maintain or improve his health. When a family focuses on what is "wrong" with the other (such as being homosexual) and tries to "fix" the other, they will induce anxiety. This leads to the development of symptoms in the family member who is singled out and most allergic to the anxiety (Maloney-Schara 1987, 2–5).

The therapist making use of family systems theory needs to be particularly sensitive to the probability of an emotional cut-off in the FWA. The male homosexual PHIV+, PWARC, and especially the PWA face a life-threatening disease with more psychosocial ramifications than any other modern illness. Therefore, his needs may be so extensive that the only system that could possibly help him address them would be his family. Even with a well-developed support system comprised of helpers from the social, legal, medical, educational, political, and religious systems, the PWA needs his family to help him deal with this crisis. His family is the first line of support and the only system with the potential strength to help him connect to other helpers. Therein lies the importance of this intervention, for knowledge of family systems theory can help the PWA, PWARC, or PHIV+ to bridge the cut-off from his family of origin.

Chapter 6

A Case Study

The case of Alex illustrates many of the elements involved in the family systems theory approach to family therapy. The story of a brief portion of his therapy shows how one confronts these dynamics of a family system in working with a person and a family with AIDS.

Alex is a twenty-nine-year-old homosexual man with AIDS. He was diagnosed one year ago when he was hospitalized with an almost fatal case of Pneumocystis carinii pneumonia. After his diagnosis, Alex returned to his home city to be closer to his family and, for the first time in their three-year relationship, took up residence with his lover Sebastiano. Alex recently quit his full-time job because it was too time consuming, tiring, and stressful. Although he works in the same industry, his present job is only part-time and gives him more opportunity to rest and exercise, things he takes very seriously. Alex is a very thoughtful young man who began therapy years ago when he first "came out" in 1984.

Alex comes from a large Polish-American family. Both his parents are the first generation of their respective families to be born in this country. All of his grandparents emigrated to the United States at about the same time and both families grew up in a very ethnic, Roman Catholic neighborhood. Alex was the first-born son, although his birth was preceded by two other pregnancies. His mother lost those children at childbirth. They were both boys. Alex was the object of a great deal of attention; he inherited his father's name as well as the very high expectations of his parents. Less than two years later Alex's sister Stephanie was born and then, seven years later, Elizabeth. Unfortunately, just a year and a half later, Elizabeth died of a congenital heart defect.

Both of Alex's parents, Alexander and Mary, are highly responsible, hardworking people. During their marriage, Mary and Alexander cared for both of their mothers when they became invalids. They also cared for Mary's sister's children when she was seriously sick, and Alexander's brother's children when his wife committed suicide. However, when Mary needed to be hospitalized, Alex and Stephanie were sent to two of Mary's girlfriends' homes rather than to any of the relatives.

Mary was the first in her family of origin to earn a college education. Currently, Alexander is finishing his bachelor's degree while Mary is working on her master's. Alexander was the first one in his family of origin to own his own home. Both Mary and Alexander received very little nurturing from their parents, and, when asked, describe their needs for affection and attention in stoic terms.

The last significant character in this web of relationships is Alex's lover, Sebastiano. Sebastiano is the first born of nine children and the only male. Born in Palermo, Sicily, Sebastiano was raised in a traditional peasant family. While he was in junior college, he "came out" to his mother who told him he must leave the house as soon as possible. A few days later Sebastiano went to live with an older man who was gay, and, shortly after that, he arranged to leave Sicily for the United States.

Individual Therapy

I became acquainted with Alex through a family support group in which his parents were participating. At the time Alex was seeing another counselor, a therapist he felt was a very kind person, but one who was unaware of the issues that were going on in his life and in his family. He made arrangements to terminate with that counselor and began weekly individual therapy with me. Some of the concerns that Alex expressed in his first individual sessions were (a) anger at his family of origin for excluding Sebastiano from the family; (b) distance from his family that began when he moved out as a teenager and got progressively worse, culminating in his moving to a distant city; and (c) his need to have a safe place to deal with the pressures of being a person with AIDS as well as his fear of losing control of his life to the disease.

In our second individual session, I explained the family systems theory approach in considerable detail. I told Alex that I would like to meet with his family of origin and him as well as with Sebastiano. Although Alex balked at the idea, he did agree that someday he might be willing to bring Sebastiano in for family counseling. However, at this point he was not ready.

An issue that has been a constant theme in our individual work is Alex's cut-off relationship with his family and his effort to resolve it. Alex's cut-off seemed to progress by degrees; first, when he moved out of the house after high school graduation; second, when he flunked out of college; and third, when he moved to another city and maintained only token contact with his parents. Interestingly, the farther away from home Alex got, the more he drank and acted impulsively in his relationships with other men. In many ways, what Alex did to his parents is quite similar to what his father and mother did to the remainder of their families. Alexander has little or no relationship with his older sister and his oldest brother, while Mary has so little contact with her brother and sister that she often says, "I have no family, that's why I want us to get along better. I don't want my kids to have to go through what I am going through."

Early in his therapy Alex confessed that he thought that running away was the best way to deal with all the feelings he had about his parents. He would often justify the distance between them and himself by quipping, "out of sight, out of mind." Alex especially felt this way about his mother because he had the most contact and conflict with her as the child-raiser of the family. Fortunately, Alex readily admitted that his behavior was counterproductive, and he was willing to admit that he carried this behavior from his relationship to his parents to his relationship with his lover. Alex is willing to reestablish individual relationships with his mother and father in an attempt to get some of his emotional needs met there. In one individual session, Alex talked warmly about going out to dinner with his father and his lover when his mother was at a meeting. Although it was not the most comfortable experience, they all had the opportunity to talk to each other in a civilized and kind way. Alex began to realize that his father was not such a bad guy, that he had some of his own unresolved issues to work on, and that he was not as homophobic as he appeared to be. Alex became the catalyst that got his entire family of origin into family therapy.

It will be important to nurture their developing relationship both in individual and family counseling. Reconnecting is also a goal for Alex and his mother. Although she can be very critical of Alex and seems to argue with him more than she does with anyone, they are talking more often and change seems to be taking place.

The issue of control will probably always be a major part of the work Alex needs to do in therapy. As developed in chapter 2, loss of control over one's life is a devastating stressor on the person with AIDS. Alex insists on taking excellent care of his health. Although there is alcohol abuse everywhere in his extended family, Alex has managed to swear off all drinking. He works out vigorously six times a week, even when he is feeling sick. Although he is eligible for disability, he insists on working part-time so he will not be too much of a burden on society. Alex is adamantly opposed to asking for any help from his parents, especially financial help. One day in individual therapy, he was complaining about how bad he felt because Sebastiano had to assume so much of the financial responsibility for their relationship. When I asked if he could turn to his parents for help, he responded quickly and sharply, "No, no, no, no, no!" Alex wants to control his health and life without any outside support. As the therapeutic process continues, we hope we will be able to temper some of his resistance by helping him see where it comes from in his family and how it contradicts his eagerness to be helpful to other people.

The life-threatening diagnosis of AIDS will be the constant issue in Alex's therapy. The psychosocial pressures that this disease puts on a person are enough to challenge even the most differentiated person. Alex and I will have to continue to monitor his thinking system so that it does not become flooded by his feeling system, and when it does, we will have to work to keep it in balance. Some of the issues that remain a constant threat to this balance are anger, fear, and loss.

Couple Therapy

Alex's relationship with Sebastiano became so conflictual that they began couple counseling with me. I interpreted this as a step closer to working with the entire family of origin, Sebastiano included. For the first two months they met with me every week, and then we scheduled our meetings every other week. One of the issues that brought Alex and Sebastiano into couple counseling was their need for belonging: Sebastiano's need to belong to Alex's family and Alex's need to belong to Sebastiano's family. For Sebastiano, this was precipitated by his fear of abandonment, as he said:

> Who will take care of me if Alex dies and I get sick? My family is thousands of miles away and they don't accept me for who I am. When Alex was in Houston on his deathbed, *I* was the one who took care of him *and* I took care of his mother! She never once asked me how I was feeling. A gay man always has to compete with his lover's mother.

Alex felt the same pressure, only for different reasons. It seems that Sebastiano is very secretive about Alex with his family and very secretive about his family with Alex. Alex feels that Sebastiano is ashamed of him or that he is not good enough for Sebastiano to want to share with his family in Sicily.

Sebastiano comes from a system that is full of emotional cutoffs and secrecy, problems that appear to be exacerbated by his Sicilian heritage. Like Alex, Sebastiano knows very little or nothing about his father's or mother's family. He talks about his extended family in terms of myths and rumors, which symbolized the distance and the mystery that characterize relationships in his family.

When Alex learned how Sebastiano's family was riddled with secrecy and homophobia, it became easier for him to understand why Sebastiano did not want him to go to Sicily with him and why Sebastiano handled it the way he did. They discussed the issue rationally and resolved to pay more attention to each other's family background and to try not to duplicate family issues (such as secrecy and shame) in their relationship.

Family Therapy

The frequency of our individual and couple sessions were reduced when Alex's family of origin began coming in for therapy as a group. This included Alex, his mother, Mary, his father, Alexander, and his sister, Stephanie. Sebastiano and Alex realized that, unfortunately, we would not be able to include Sebastiano in Alex's family's therapy at this point. Both Sebastiano and Alex felt that if someone were there whom the family did not consider a "real" part of the family, they would be more resistant than they usually were when talking about difficult, personal issues.

One of the most powerful issues in this family's therapy is Alex's relationship to his family of origin and their relationship to his lover. It is important to view the family of a homosexual man with AIDS in a way that is broad enough to include his "family of choice," an intimate group of homosexual friends. This "family" includes the entire kinship network of at least three generations both as it currently exists and as it has evolved. It is much easier to see how the family projection process is at work from this point of view.

The family projection process is at work in Alex's family. Both of Alex's parents have distant, conflictual relationships with most members of their families of origin. For example, Mary is significantly cut-off from her sister and brother. She only sees them when there is a death or a wedding in the family, and then she attends begrudgingly. On more than one occasion in family therapy, Mary claimed to be closer to Alexander's brother Bruce than to her siblings. Once she said, "I don't have a family except for Alexander's brother, Bruce." This situation might lead one to believe that Alexander is very close to his family, especially his brother Bruce. However, that is far from the truth. Alexander thinks that his two oldest siblings are "flakes" and describes his relationship with his brother Bruce as very close. Yet he only sees Bruce two or three times a year and rarely communicates at other times. According to Alex, the only time they really have anything to say to each other is when they both have had too much to drink.

It also appears that Alex's parents have never fully grieved the death of their youngest daughter. These factors help to create a system in which the unresolved issues of the parents (such as cut-offs, unmet dependency needs) are passed on to one of the children to be resolved. The child to receive that projection was Alex, who was perceived as a "sissy" because he liked to play house and was not adept at playing some sports. It was not until his high school years that Alex was able to make his mark as a track star; by that time the die was cast and the projection process was already in operation.

One of the ways that Alex's family's unresolved issues get projected onto Alex is in his family's unwillingness to accept themselves and support each other. Both Mary and Alexander had very few of their childhood needs filled by their parents. Now they are very concerned with Alex's health and future but, at the same time, they cannot give Alex what he needs just as their parents could not give them what they needed. Alexander and Mary often state how much they love their children, but when their children ask for the acceptance that comes from love, Alexander and Mary cannot seem to understand what they want. In some ways they are all playing a game: The parents say they want to give their children what they need, but they do not listen to their requests. The children try to tell the parents what they want, but when the parents try to respond, the children resent it. A good example is Alex's longing for his father's acceptance and affection. However, when his father tries to be affectionate by hugging him hello, Alex rejects this fatherly affection and complains, "He didn't give it to me when I wanted it; now that he wants it I don't because it's phony." From a therapeutic point of view, I am trying to use the crisis of AIDS as a catalyst to break the family rule that states that no one should ever ask for help because if he or she does ask he or she will not get it. Perhaps we will be able to use the pressure that AIDS exerts on a family to move them away from this circular law and invite them to realize that the entire family unit needs to make some radical changes in the way it does business.

Another family issue that gets projected onto Alex is the issue of sexuality. For Alexander and Mary sexuality is "dirty," and the messages they send to Alex are homo-negative if not homophobic. Subsequently, Alex's relationship with his lover is an easy target for this projection process. Therefore, any effort to do family therapy without involving Sebastiano in some way would be a job poorly done. Sebastiano, his family of origin, and their issues are also integral parts of what is going on in this "extended family."

Alex's diagnosis of AIDS needs to be viewed as a total family problem. If not, Alex's illness may be treated in isolation from his relationships when, in reality, his AIDS has a great effect on all his relationships and all his relationships have a great effect on his AIDS.

Alex's family responds stoically in most affective issues. For instance, in one therapy session Alex told how his father never cried at his baby sister's funeral, and yet now his father repeatedly mentions how I hugged Alex at the funeral of Bill, another young man whose family attended the family support group. Alex's family's stoicism and rigid interpretation of their faith also color the way they deal with sexuality. At another therapy session, Alex related how he was publicly humiliated by his mother when, at the age of five, she found him with his hands in his pants touching his genitals. As Alex grew older, these attitudes easily developed into homophobia. Alex vividly remembers how his Uncle Bruce would regularly ridicule homosexual people and how, especially when his father and uncle were drinking, homosexuals were the brunt of their humor and sarcasm.

Mary's high expectations of her children and her severity toward them can be traced to her family of origin, a dysfunctional family. Although second youngest by birth order, Mary fulfilled the position of the highly responsible child in her family. Mary's father died of cirrhosis of the liver due to alcohol abuse when she was only six. During that same year Mary's baby sister Stephanie and her highly responsible grandmother also died. Subsequently, Mary's grandfather took over the male responsibilities of the family. Within a few years, Mary took over the female responsibilities because Mary's mother was also an irresponsible chronic alcoholic. Mary's responsibility was fine-tuned by her grandfather, a hardworking and dedicated man who was her salvation. Mary internalized his values and became a hardworking, highly responsible young girl. Because her grandfather was able but not willing to send her to a private Catholic high school, Mary got a job as a nanny and paid her own way through high school and college, a feat that neither her brother nor sister accomplished.

Alexander also contributes to the responsibility issue in two significant ways. First, because of his hardworking nature he always held two jobs, and now that his children are on their own, he is finishing his B.S. degree in night school. As a result of this, he never had much to do with the rearing of the children. In many ways he abdicated most of his authority to his wife, while supporting her emotional involvement with the children. Second, he too inherited a strong sense of responsibility from his family of origin. His oldest brother was blind, never married, and died at an early age. His oldest sister has a long history of alcohol abuse and institutionalizations for emotional problems; and his next oldest brother is an artist who never seemed to have much of a sense of responsibility. Consequently, Alexander and his younger brother Bruce became highly motivated and successful people.

Alexander and Mary appear to have brought very high expectations of themselves into their relationship and transmitted those expectations to their children in subtle ways. Some of the messages that get delivered are: you must get a good education; you must surpass your parents; you must not think too much of yourselves; you should never get too interested in sexuality; you must make us proud of you by being ideal children; and, possibly the most powerful message, you must take care of our unmet childhood needs but we cannot be direct about what those needs are and we will probably reject your offer if you do try to meet them. Alex internalized these messages because of his birth order, a position that was exacerbated by the fact that his first two siblings were boys who died in childbirth. This message became even more powerful when Elizabeth died and left Stephanie the only girl in the family. Now that Alex's life is threatened by

AIDS, Stephanie lives in constant fear that Alex will die and leave her the only surviving child and the only recipient of the expectations that would have been spread out over five children.

The atmosphere becomes even more intense when Alex's lover Sebastiano is included. Sebastiano's birthday is Christmas Eve. What to do on Christmas Eve became a powerful question for Alex and Sebastiano. Since Sebastiano had not seen his family in over six years and was significantly cut-off from them, he projected many of his needs onto Alex and his family. Alex's family was not only relatively homophobic but had always reserved Christmas Eve for their family of origin to gather in memory of baby Elizabeth. Sebastiano now presented a double threat to Alex's family. Of course Alex felt caught between a rock and a hard place. On one side he had his family and their unconscious need to mourn the death of their last born; on the other hand, he had his lover who had no family to support him on his birthday and was connected to a substitute family whose homophobia kept him at a great distance. Add to this Alexander's and Mary's suspicion that Sebastiano was the one who infected Alex, and all the elements for a disaster are present. In both individual and couple counseling, we used this dilemma to de-triangle Alex from his unfortunate position of being caught between his parents and his lover. As therapy continued, Alex resolved to sit down his mother and father and tell them that Christmas Eve was also Sebastiano's birthday and that he wanted to celebrate that day with him because he was so far away from home. He also told them that he wanted to celebrate Christmas Eve with his parents and sister as long as his lover was welcomed. Alex, however, refused to be triangled in between his parents and Sebastiano, so he suggested that his parents call Sebastiano and personally invite him to the celebration. If they could not do that and if Sebastiano would not cooperate, then Alex would spend Christmas Eve alone. Sebastiano agreed to this plan while they were both at a pre-Christmas Eve couple session. However, Sebastiano made is perfectly clear that if invited, he would arrive for dinner at 5:30 P.M. and leave at 8:30 P.M., with or without Alex.

At my next one-to-one session with Alex, which happened three days after Christmas, I found out some remarkable facts. A few days after the pre-Christmas couple session Alex had a long talk with his parents. Consequently, Alex's mother called Sebastiano and invited him for Christmas Eve dinner. On the day of Christmas Eve, Alex served Sebastiano breakfast in bed and made him a special birthday cake. They spent the entire day together until 5:30 P.M. when they went to Alex's parents for dinner. Sebastiano had a wonderful time and stayed until 11:45 P.M. Sebastiano and Alex left just in time to attend Midnight Mass together, and afterward joined some friends to have a drink and continue to celebrate Sebastiano's birthday at a local gay bar. The next day Alex drove Sebastiano to the airport for his first trip back to Sicily in eight years. Sebastiano called Alex every other day of his ten-day trip.

This sequence of events would be a wonderful holiday story with a happy ending if it were not a classic example of how the deleterious effects of the family projection process continue to operate. Just as Alex began to extricate himself from the triangle between his parents and his lover, it appears that Stephanie may be taking his place. Despite repeated telephone requests, Stephanie refused to leave her friends at the bar where she worked and attend the annual Christmas Eve dinner. On the day set aside to memorialize her infant sister's death (and almost one year since her brother was diagnosed with AIDS and was told he had about a year to live), Stephanie could not bear to be with the family that might put her into a position she found intolerable. Her refusal to attend the Christmas Eve dinner started a new crisis for the family, and offered them a new focus for their dysfunctional attention.

Shortly after Christmas the family agreed to start coming to therapy together. Within the first session the issue of expectations came up with a vengeance. Despite Alexander's rationalizations and Mary's refusal to see that she and her husband are highly motivated people with high expectations of themselves and their children, Alex and Stephanie, but especially Stephanie, insisted that they were demanding parents. Stephanie recounted that she always felt like a failure because she was not a good student, because she could not get a good job, and because she had a series of unfortunate and painful relationships with young men. Using examples from her childhood and from her recent past, Stephanie tried to show her parents how demanding they were even though they did not intend to be that way. It seemed to me that as Alex was extricating himself from a system that needed a scapegoat, Stephanie was putting up a valiant effort to make sure she was not going to be Alex's replacement. Denial seemed to be the defense of the day. Both Alexander and Mary kept protesting that they were not overly responsible people who demanded too much of their children. When asked to share things about their positions in their respective families of origin, both Alexander and Mary resisted and resented any implication that they were high achievers who did what they set out to do. Alexander would always react defensively, by quipping, "Why are we talking about me? I don't want to be in the limelight. I came here to talk about Alex." When I would point out their accomplishments, they would both protest that they only did what everyone else in their generation had to do. Both Mary and Alexander reacted as if they were being blamed for something despite all my efforts to lead the conversation in terms of the entire family and not just one "identified patient."

An important part of our family work is my constant reminder that these are not issues of blame but rather a function of the family projection process. In other words, it is not Mary's and Alexander's fault that they have these high expectations, but rather it is the way the family does business based on the way their families did business. Within moments of this reminder, Alexander reacted somewhat defensively by declaring that he never meant to hurt his children, he just wanted them to be happy, to settle down, get married, and have kids. We used his very normal expectations to show him how it played out in a negative way in this family. When Alex hears such messages from his father, he begins to feel that he has failed his father because he is gay and will not have children. One of the therapeutic goals will be to show this family how they unconsciously and unintentionally communicate unresolved issues (such as high expectations) from one generation to another.

Homophobia is probably the second most powerful issue in this family's therapy. In many ways, Alex's Uncle Bruce has become the symbol of the family's inability to accept Alex as a homosexual man, let alone accept Sebastiano as his lover and a member of their extended family. Bruce is not only Alexander's closest sibling, but Mary has an enormous investment in him as well because she is so distant from her own family. Unfortunately, Bruce is very homophobic. Although Alex always looked up to his uncle before, he is becoming less tolerant of his uncle now that he is spending so much time trying to understand himself in the context of his family.

Recently Alexander felt a need to tell his brother about Alex's diagnosis. So, in one fell swoop, Bruce found out that his favorite nephew was both gay and suffering from AIDS, an excellent example of the double-barrel effect (cf. chapter 3). In reporting a recent phone conversation with his Uncle Bruce, Alex recounted how Bruce ended up saying, "Alex, we love you." Alex countered by saying, "Yeah, sure."

Fortunately, some inroads have been made. Alexander and Mary regularly attend a family support group for mothers, fathers, sisters, brothers, wives, husbands, and lovers of people with AIDS. A good illustration of how this experience has been desensitizing for them happened at the family support group Christmas party at my home. Because I was busy in the kitchen, I asked Mary, a very hospitable woman, to act as hostess. This meant that she would have to introduce everyone to those who were joining us for the first time. These guests included three gay men whose lovers were regular members of the group. Probably for the first time in her life, Mary went around a crowded room saying, "Ethel, I'd like you to meet John's lover, Jeff." Later that same evening when we were sharing appetizers, Alexander commented on how delicious one of the hors d'oeuvres was. I told him that Ed's lover, Mike, made them. He turned to his wife and said, "Mary, you have to taste these. Ed's lover, Mike, made them. They're delicious." Alex, who was a guest of his parents, stood in the corner and watched all of this happen.

Currently, Alex's family is still in therapy, and, although a final resolution may be far off, they have made a serious commitment to become a healthier family. Alex claims to have more control over the disease than ever before. He is taking excellent care of his health as testified by his rededication to wholistic medicine. He feels less stressful and claims to have more energy. To his parents' surprise and pleasure, Alex is applying to local colleges in an attempt to fulfill his dreams of finishing a bachelor's degree in physical therapy. He and Sebastiano are getting along better than ever and are dealing with their health and financial problems by talking as openly as they can although, at times, the burden of AIDS makes communicating difficult. As for Alex's family, the process goes slowly but in the right direction. They are communicating more honestly than ever before and, although their communications are often conflictual, they are beginning to recognize what is going on in their family without blaming themselves or one of their children.

Working with Alex, Sebastiano, and their families is an important lesson in differentiation.

Chapter 7

CONCLUSION

The story of Alex makes it extremely clear that one cannot counsel an individual with AIDS without dealing with the family in some sense. Frequently, when a young adult is confronted with a life-threatening disease, the family of origin plays an important part in the emotional and financial support of that person. In the case of the gay person with AIDS, it is very common for the patient to return to the home of his parents for support. In such a situation, the family of origin can be on the front line of care. Therefore, in addition to pastoral care with the person with AIDS or AIDS Related Complex (ARC) or who tests positive for human immunodeficiency virus (HIV+), there is a great opportunity and challenge for pastoral care and counseling with the family of that person. Family systems theory provides many insights for meeting that challenge.

Pastoral counseling and care for the family can become more important if the PWA, PWARC, or PHIV+ is totally alienated from the church. There may be cases where the PWA does not want the services of the minister. However, under such circumstances, the pastoral counselor or caregiver should not conclude that the family of the PWA, PWARC, or PHIV+ does not need his or her services. Mothers, fathers, sisters, brothers, lovers, etc., may have a strong need to speak with a church or religious representative. The fact that a pastoral counselor or caregiver would make his or her services available could be perceived as a confirmation of God's acceptance of their suffering loved one, and perhaps even a confirmation of the church's acceptance. The family with AIDS (FWA) needs such a person to help them overcome the pressures caused by alienation, secrecy, guilt, fear, shame, or perceived family failure. Also, service to the FWA is an excellent way to break the ice with the gay PWA, PWARC, or PHIV +. If the patient sees that the pastoral counselor or caregiver is loyal, nonjudgmental, dedicated, and concerned about his family, it is only one more step for him to see that the same applies to him. The family can be both an end and a means to an end.

The pastoral counselor or caregiver can be especially useful if the family is angry at the PWA, PWARC, or PHIV +. The family may feel that their son or brother has been irresponsible, unfaithful (that is, to the lover), sinful, or an undeserved burden. The diagnosis of AIDS, ARC, or HIV + can bring to the surface the family's unresolved feelings of homophobia; or rage and rejection may surface when the family finds out that their son is gay *and* has a life-threatening disease. If the patient has a lover, the family may not know how to deal with him, or, worse yet, presume that he was the one who infected their son. It is not difficult to imagine the horrible scenarios that could develop in such a case, including the demand that the PWA, PWARC, or PHIV + make a choice between his family of origin and his family of choice (Shelp & Sunderland 1987, 46). The family of origin, potentially the best equipped and most appropriate system that could be available to help the PWA, PWARC, or PHIV +, could easily become his worst enemy. The pastoral counselor or caregiver must be aware of the potential for good and evil that exists in any family. By his or her acceptance of the PWA, PWARC, or PHIV +, the pastoral counselor or caregiver can model for the family a more appropriate response to their wounded son or brother. Or, by allowing the FWA to vent some of their rage at him, the minister could lead them down the path of acceptance.

Religious tradition . . . provides a bridge by which the individual is able to tie together new, and, in the case of AIDS, cataclysmic information with coping mechanisms and personal family traditions to help a patient understand and accept. This bridge is not simply one way. Families and significant others also search for these bridges so they can begin to assimilate and respond to new and threatening information (Marshall 1987, 18).

The pastoral counselor or caregiver can be of invaluable service as a representative of the religious tradition and a bridge builder. Although there are no easy answers to the pastoral counseling and care of the PWA, PWARC, or PHIV +, experience offers us some valuable insights. It would be remarkable if the pastoral counselor or caregiver could be part of the process that helps the PWA, PWARC, or PHIV + say: "I never could have grown in this way if it hadn't been for AIDS."

A PERSONAL EPILOGUE

I know many people with AIDS. They are clients I see for psychotherapy, patients I visit at the AIDS clinic, and people I serve dinner to at the "PWA Supper Club." They are, almost to a person, insightful men and women who have an understanding of life far beyond their years. I suspect their wisdom comes from their role as the lepers of the twentieth century, for almost all of them have extracted something of great value from this crisis.

I am grateful to them for everything they have taught me about life and death and life everlasting.

I am proud of them for their bravery in demanding their rights as citizens, humans, and children of God.

I am in awe of them for the patience and understanding they exhibit in the face of rash judgment and sarcasm.

Finally, I am moved to tears each time one of them asks me to celebrate his or her funeral service. It is a pain that I already know too well, a pain that, along with AIDS, I pray will go away very soon.

BIBLIOGRAPHY

Abbott, W., ed. *The Documents of Vatican II*. New York: Guild Press, 1966.

Baum, R. "The Molecular Biology." *Chemical and Engineering News* 65 (1987): 21.

Bondings, a newsletter of New Ways Ministry. 10 (Winter): 1987–88.

Bradley, J. "The Bittersweet Life of Jimmy Holloran." *The Family Therapy Networker*, January/February 1988, 45–89.

Bowen, M. *Family Therapy in Clinical Practice*. Northvale, N.J.: Jason Aronson, 1978.

Brown, H. *Familiar Faces, Hidden Lives: The Story of Homosexual Men in America Today*. New York: Harcourt Brace Jovanovich, 1976.

Declaration on Certain Questions Concerning Sexual Ethics. Washington, D.C.: Office of Publishing and Promotion Services, United States Catholic Conference, 1975.

Demartini, R. "A Fool's Death." *Communication Ministry, Inc. Journal 10* (1987): 9–12.

Dunphy, R. "AIDS and Spirituality." *FOCUS, A Guide to AIDS Research* 3 (1987): 1–2.

Dupree, D. and G. Margo, "Homophobia, AIDS and the Health Care Professional." *FOCUS, A Guide to AIDS Research*, January 1988, 1–2.

Economic Justice for All. Washington, D.C.: Office of Publishing and Promotion Services, United States Catholic Conference, 1986.

Flynn, E. *AIDS, a Catholic Call for Compassion.* Kansas City: Sheed & Ward, 1986.

Fortunato, J. *Embracing the Exile: Healing Journeys for Gay Christians.* San Francisco: Harper & Row, 1982.

Fortunato, J. "AIDS: The Plague That Lays Waste at Noon." *The Witness* 68 (1985): 6–9.

Framo, J. L. *Explorations in Marital and Family Therapy.* New York: Springer Publishing, 1978.

Friedman, E. *Generation to Generation.* New York: The Guilford Press, 1985.

Frutchey, C. "Homophobia in AIDS Education: Counterproductive to prevention." *FOCUS, A Guide to AIDS Research,* January 1988, 3–4.

Gallagher, J. *Voices of Strength and Hope for a Friend with AIDS.* Kansas City: Sheed & Ward, 1987.

Gilbert, J. "Coming to Terms." *The Family Therapy Networker,* January/February 1988, 42–43, 81.

The Gospel Alive. St. Louis: The Catholic Health Association of the United States, 1988.

Goldenberg, I. and H. Goldenberg. *Family Therapy: An Overview.* Monterey, Calif.: Brooks/Cole Publishing Co., 1980.

Gramick, J., ed. *Homosexuality and the Catholic Church.* Mt. Rainier, Md.: New Ways Ministry, 1983.

Guerin, P. J. *Family Therapy.* New York: Gardner Press, 1976.

Guggenbuhl-Craig, A. *Marriage Dead or Alive.* Dallas: Spring Publications, 1977.

Gurman, A. and D. Kniskern., eds. *Handbook of Family Therapy.* New York: Brunner/Mazel, 1981.

Haber, R. "Friends in Family Therapy: Use of a Neglected Resource." *Family Process* 26 (1987): 269–282.

Haley, J. *Changing Families.* New York: Grune & Stratton, 1971.

Halpern, H. M. *Cutting Loose.* Toronto: Bantam Books, 1976.

Harvey, J. "Homosexuality." In *The New Catholic Encyclopedia.* New York: McGraw-Hill, 1967. 7:116–19.

Hanigan, J. *Homosexuality: The Test Case for Christian Sexual Ethics.* New York: Paulist Press, 1988.

Hansen, J. *Sexual Issues in Family Therapy.* Rockville, Md.: Aspen Systems Corporation, 1983.

Hoffman, L. *Foundations of Family Therapy.* New York: Basic Books, 1981.

Horne, A. M., and M. M. Ohlsen. *Family Counseling and Therapy.* Itasca, Ill.: F. E. Peacock Publishers, 1982.

Howells, J., and W. Guirguis. *The Family and Schizophrenia.* Madison, Conn.: International Universities Press, 1984.

Humphrey, F. G. *Marital Therapy.* Englewood Cliffs, N.J.: Prentice-Hall, 1983.

Kerr, M., and M. Bowen. *Family Evaluation: An Approach Based on Bowen Theory.* New York: W. W. Norton & Co., 1988.

Kosnik, A., et al. *Human Sexuality.* New York: Paulist Press, 1977.

Lancaster, M. "AIDS and the Family." Seminar paper submitted to the Faculty of the Graduate School of the University of Maryland, 1987.

Letter to the Bishops of the Catholic Church on the Pastoral Care of Homosexual Persons. Washington, D.C.: Office of Publishing and Promotion Services, United States Catholic Conference, 1986.

Lewis, C. "The Impact of AIDS on Medicine." *FOCUS, A Guide to AIDS Research,* March 1988, 1–2.

Lieberman, S. *Transgenerational Family Therapy.* London: Croom Helm, 1979.

The Link. Council for Health and Human Service Ministries, Lancaster, Pa. Vol. 4, no. 1 (January 1987).

"Living with AIDS. A Guide to the Legal Problems of People with AIDS." New York: Lambda Legal Defense and Education Fund, Inc, 1987.

"The Loss of Leaving Home." *Family Therapy Today,* November 1986, 5–6.

Lynch, B. "Jimmy: Duine le Dia." *Communication Ministry, Inc. Journal* 10 (1987): 15–17.

Maloney-Schara, A. "Towards a Bowen Family Systems Perspective: AIDS in the Family." Presentation to Biofeedback Society of Washington, D.C. and Maryland, October 10, 1987.

"The Many Faces of AIDS." Washington, D.C.: Office of Publishing and Promotion Services, United States Catholic Conference, 1987.

Marshall, T. "Pastoral Counseling, Care Involves Family and Medical Staff." *AIDS Patient Care*, September 1987:18–21.

McBrien, R. P. *Catholicism*. Minneapolis: Winston Press, 1987.

McGoldrick, M. *Ethnicity and Family Therapy*. New York: The Guilford Press, 1982.

McGoldrick, M. *Genograms in Family Assessment*. New York: W. W. Norton and Co. 1985.

McNeil, J. *The Church and the Homosexual*. 3d ed. Boston: Beacon Press, 1988.

Meyer, M. "The Catholic Church and AIDS." *America*, June 1986, 512–13.

Minuchin, S. *Families and Family Therapy*. Cambridge: Harvard Univ. Press, 1974.

"A Model Based Estimate of the Mean Incubation Period for AIDS in Homosexual Men." *Science* 240 (1988): 1333–35.

Murphy, D. "Third Thursday Profession Meeting, AIDS and the Family." *Family Center Report*, 9 (Winter 1988): 3–5.

Nagy, Boszormenyi- I. and B. Krasner, *Between Give and Take*. New York: Runner/Mazel, 1986.

Napier, A. Y. *The Family Crucible*. New York: Harper and Row, 1978.

Nichols, M. *Family Therapy: Concepts and Methods*. New York: Gardner Press, 1984.

Noer, H. *Family Center Report*. Department of Psychiatry, Georgetown University School of Medicine. Vol. 9, no. 1 (Winter 1988).

Palazzoli, M. S. *Paradox and Counter Paradox*. New Jersey: Jason Aronson, 1978.

Paolino, T., and B. McCrady. *Marriage and Marital Therapy*. New York: Brunner/Mazel, 1978.

Patten, John. "AIDS and the Gay Couple." *The Family Therapy Networker*. (January/February 1988): 37–39.

Patton, C. *Sex and Germs*. Boston: South End Press, 1985.

Peabody, Barbara. *The Screaming Room*. San Diego: Oak Tree Publications, Inc., 1986.

Quinn, F. To the people of the Catholic Diocese of Sacramento concerning the Christian response in caring for our brothers and sisters with AIDS. May 21, 1986.

Quinn, J. R. "The AIDS Crisis: A Pastoral Response." *America*, June 1986, 505–6.

Scanzoni, L. D., and J. Scanzoni. *Men, Women and Change*. New York: McGraw Hill, 1981.

Selwyn, P. *AIDS: What Is Now Known*. New York: HP Publishing, 1986.

Shelp, E., and R. Sunderland. *AIDS and the Church*. Philadelphia: Westminster Press, 1987.

Shenson, D. "When Fear Conquers All." *The New York Times Magazine*, February 1988, 36–48.

Simos, B. "Loss and Grief in Family Therapy." *Family Therapy Today* 1 (1986): 1–2, 6–7.

Stulz, J. "Towards a Spirituality for Victims of AIDS." *America*, June 1986, 509–11.

Umbarger, C. C. *Structural Family Therapy*. New York: Grune and Straton, 1983.

U.S. Department of Health and Human Services. *Understanding AIDS*. Rockville, Md: HHS Publication No. (CDC) HHS-88-8404.

Walker, G. "AIDS and Family Therapy." *Family Therapy Today* 2 (April 1987): 1–2, 6–7.

Walker, G. "AIDS and Family Therapy, Part II." *Family Therapy Today* 2 (June 1987b): 1–7.

Walker, G. "An AIDS Journal." *The Family Therapy Networker*, January/February 1988, 20–32, 76–79.

Walsh, F. *Normal Family Processes*. New York: Guilford Press, 1982.

Waltzlawick, P. *Change*. New York: W. W. Norton, 1974.

Woititz, J. *Struggle for . . . Intimacy*. Pompano Beach: Health Communications, Inc., 1985.

Wynn, J. C. *Family Therapy in Pastoral Ministry*. San Francisco: Harper & Row, 1982.